SUPER FITNESS BEYOND VITAMINS

The Bible of Super Supplements

SUPER FITNESS BEYOND VITAMINS

The Bible of Super Supplements

by
Michael E. Rosenbaum, M.D.
and
Dominick Bosco

NAL BOOKS

NEW AMERICAN LIBRARY

NEW YORK AND SCARBOROUGH, ONTARIO

Published simultaneously in Canada by The New American Library
of Canada Limited

 NAL BOOKS TRADEMARK REG. U.S. PAT. OFF. AND FOREIGN COUNTRIES
REGISTERED TRADEMARK—MARCA REGISTRADA
HECHO EN HARRISONBURG, VA., U.S.A.

SIGNET, SIGNET CLASSIC, MENTOR, ONYX, PLUME,
MERIDIAN and NAL BOOKS are published *in the United States* by
NAL PENGUIN INC., 1633 Broadway, New York, New York 10019,
in Canada by The New American Library of Canada Limited,
81 Mack Avenue, Scarborough, Ontario M1L 1M8

Library of Congress Cataloging-in-Publication Data

Rosenbaum, Michael E.
  Super fitness beyond vitamins.

  1. Dietary supplements. 2. Physical fitness.
3. Health. I. Bosco, Dominick. II. Title. [DNLM:
1. Physical Fitness—popular works. 2. Vitamins—
popular works. QU 160 R8127s]
RA784.R66 1987   613.2   87-7707
ISBN 0-453-00545-4

Designed by Julian Hamer

First Printing, August, 1987

1 2 3 4 5 6 7 8 9

PRINTED IN THE UNITED STATES OF AMERICA

We dedicate this book to
Linus Pauling and Abram Hoffer, M.D.,
in appreciation of their genius,
courage, and conviction in exploring and
advocating optimum intake of nutrients
for better health.

ACKNOWLEDGMENTS

I would like to express my appreciation to:

The Huxley Institute, for its dedicated support and promotion of nutritional medicine;

Richard Kunin, M.D., who gave me my start in nutritional medicine;

Lorna Creveling, whose courageous struggle to overcome a disabling illness continually challenges my growth as a physician;

Stephen Levine, Ph.D., my close friend, whose innovating research has had a profound impact on our appreciation of the role of antioxidants in health and disease;

Jeffrey Anderson, M.D., my colleague, from whom I have learned so much;

Andrew Kluger, for his wise counsel and support;

Sarah Gold, my beautiful sister;

Gerda Fiske, my mother-in-law, for all the happiness she has cultivated;

Christina, my wife and inspiration;

Ivory, Crystal, and Amber, for the joy only they could bring;

Sydney Rosenbaum, my recently departed father, for teaching me, in his own gentle way, the fear of God;

Anna Rosenbaum, my mother and the best cook I've ever known.

—M. E. R.

And I would like to thank the following people, without whose guidance, support, and inspiration this book would not have been possible:

Robin Rogosin, and Barbara Miller at Mrs. Gooch's, for their confirmation that this book was needed;

Janice Gallagher and Jeremy Tarcher for their initial belief in this project;

Rob Krakovitz, M.D., for introducing me to Michael Rosenbaum;

Jeff and Julie Katke of Metagenics and Bill Thompson, John Foster, and Ron Martin of Thompson's for their most generous and unconditional help with the research;

Jeff Bland, Ph.D., for his expert advice;

Dale and Silky Alexander for knowing the benefit of fish oil before everybody else;

Sandy Gooch and Harry Lederman for their hospitality, support, and love;

Hyla Cass, M.D., for sharing;

Sandra Watt, for her enthusiasm and friendship;

Carole Hall, our editor, for her steadfast belief in our book and her skillful guidance in shaping the manuscript;

Russell Galen, for his generosity and able care;

The Kostrubala Family: Tad, Teresa, Giovanna, Tadz, Christine, and Kazimir—for adopting me;

Father George and Helen Benigsen, for their prayers;

Leslie Howard Lang, my brother;

Sunny and Bonne and Teri, as always, for the joy they bring to my life;

Loretta, my sister, who inspires me with her courage and love;

Joseph Bosco, my father, for all the trips to and from the airport;

Emma Bosco, my mother, for all the vitamins and chocolate cake.

—D. B.

Contents

Introduction

by Michael E. Rosenbaum, M.D.

I believe the body has a wisdom and a power all its own and, if encouraged and supported, can heal itself.

Years ago, the stress of a demanding medical practice caught up with me. Not only was I often physically exhausted, but even normal mental processes sometimes seemed an uphill battle. Today, we would have called my condition "burnout."

To find a way to help myself, I started reading voraciously in the field of nutrition.

The changes I made in my diet and the supplements I took really worked: I started to improve. I had more energy. I looked better and better. My strength returned. My digestive disturbances disappeared. I got better.

You can't imagine what a turnaround this was for me! I began to see health and medicine in a totally different way. Mind you—it was a matter of my own health and happiness. Not only did this new knowledge make sense, but it also made me feel a lot better about myself and about the possibilities for helping people by practicing medicine.

But it would have to be a different kind of medicine.

I was convinced that nutrition could play a critical role in healing.

I transformed my own life first. After that, it was the only way I could practice medicine. I was duty-bound to use what I knew worked. Though I'm sure there are many fine physicians for whom the conventional way works, and though I use drugs and surgery when necessary, I never knew the real meaning of healing until I started practicing nutritional medicine.

When I first began practicing nutritional medicine, we had a much more limited array of nutritional tools than we do now. Over the years, we've learned more and more about how specific nutrients can help us grow stronger and healthier. There are supplements we didn't even dream about just a decade ago. This book is going to bring you up to date on what nutritional supplements can do for you, and help you design a personal program that can serve your special needs.

Introduction

by Dominick Bosco

Over the past 12 years I've worked with more than 100 physicians. I can say that all of them were sincerely devoted to helping their patients get well and stay well. Michael Rosenbaum stands out, not only because of his vast knowledge of nutrition, but also because of his deep, caring instincts. One of the hardest things about being a doctor is you must give a little of yourself to every patient. I know Michael gives more of himself than most. I have sat outside his office and watched his patients come and go. Many of them come to him because they have been unable to find help elsewhere. Michael always helps them. Now he can help you, too.

Our aims in this book are:

To present a program to guide you in the use of any and all nutritional supplements you might choose to include in your diet.

To present information on new supplements we have never seen gathered in one place—and some information we have never seen at all in a book for laypeople.

Our aim is not to take the place of good medical care. When you have a medical problem, there is no substitute for the trained eye and skilled care of a physician.

However, even the best medical care depends on the self-healing powers of the body and the will of the person to strengthen those powers. Our hope is that the information in this book will support your efforts.

As an editor of *Prevention* magazine, I had the opportunity to interview and collaborate with many physicians who were at the forefront of nutritional therapy. That's when I could see, firsthand, how the information revealed in the thousands of scientific reports was already being put to practical use in helping people get better.

I can't write about things I don't believe in. Through the years, I've tried to use my knowledge of nutrition to help myself and my friends and family live healthier and happier lives. I've written this book in that spirit, to share this information with you.

Go Beyond Vitamins!

CHAPTER
1 Your Fitness Potential in a Bold New World of Health

EVERYTIME a ship leaves on a voyage of discovery, there's an enlightened group on board bound for a peak experience. It's the same for a spaceship leaving for the moon as it was for Columbus setting sail for the New World. Some people are always ready for bold new steps.

And so it is with the new age of health. As millions of people have already discovered, each of us has the right to reach for a higher level of personal health, strength, and happiness. *Super Fitness Beyond Vitamins* will give you the means to stretch beyond arbitrary definitions of "normal" well-being, improve your mental and physical functioning, enhance your resistance to stress, achieve a better sex life, and discover a host of other benefits.

There is a growing body of evidence from research and clinical experience which says that if you're only taking vitamin–mineral supplements and ignoring certain other vital nutrients, then:

- You may not be getting all the benefits you think you are
- You may be taking too much of some substances and not enough of what you really need
- You may be missing out on many of the health benefits research and clinical experience have demonstrated for the new super supplements.

The nutrients generating the most exciting and promising news are amino acids, enzymes, bioflavonoids, essential oils, and glandulars. Our "bible" will enable you to select individual supplements to add to your already-existing program—or help you plan a new, complete supplement program, custom-designed for your own needs and specifications.

You'll learn:

What supplements can chase away fatigue

What supplements can boost professional and athletic performance to peak levels while building reserve energy

What supplements can enhance your sexual drive, potency, and fertility

What supplements will strengthen the immune system to help the body guard against infectious diseases such as herpes, flu, and possibly AIDS

What supplements may give you the benefits of an expensive European rejuvenation clinic—for 1/500 the cost

How to sharply reduce the effects of food allergies without giving up your favorite foods (which probably are the foods that cause the allergic reaction)

How to combine your supplements

What supplements to take during and after a weight-loss diet to make sure that any diet which successfully takes off pounds will do it quicker, safer, and keep them off longer

What supplements to take to maximize the efficiency of all nutrients, including those in food and in other supplements

Plus—a special bonus—seven nutrition secrets you should know

In taking you beyond vitamins, we are going to fill you in on the exciting new information about vitamins and minerals. Our goal is not to diminish the importance of these nutrients. We want to make your foundation on them strong and sure—and then take you beyond them.

Super Fitness Beyond Vitamins will give you state-of-the-art multisupplements for specific individual needs:

specifically—boosting immunity, losing weight, fighting allergies, enhancing physical, mental, and sexual performance, resisting stress, and feeling younger longer.

You will be astonished by the range of potentially effective supplements available to you.

Just as we were preparing the final draft of *Super Fitness Beyond Vitamins*, a story unfolded that perfectly illustrates the fitness benefits you can achieve with this approach to supplementation.

The story began when Helen, a thirty-four-year-old sales manager from San Francisco, came to my office (MR) complaining of severe premenstrual syndrome. Helen's general health was good, and I could see no factors in her diet that might be causing her problems. Yet, three weeks out of every month, Helen was barely able to function. In addition to having the classic symptoms of discomfort and weight gain, she admitted she also became very difficult to get along with. Despite her extreme effort to keep her irritability and other mental symptoms under control, she frequently got into arguments with customers and her employees. Since she had to deal with people almost constantly in her work, her PMS was clearly threatening her livelihood as well as her health. Helen had been to other physicians, who prescribed tranquilizers and diuretics. Neither of these drugs had worked for her.

Increasing doses of vitamins and minerals did not help, either. There was a sharp edge of disappointment in her voice as she shook her head and said, over and over, "Nothing works!"

After Helen's first visit, she called to tell me she had learned of a new supplement for PMS: anterior pituitary substance, a glandular supplement. I was skeptical, because there didn't seem to be a lot of research explaining why this supplement should work for PMS. But I also had no reason to believe that the supplement could do any harm. Since there were reports that it had helped some women, I told Helen there was no reason not to give it a try. I explained that I didn't know exactly how it might work, but that some doctors had reported that it could work. Helen said she was willing to try the supplement.

I was astonished! Helen's response to the supplement was dramatic. She was transformed! On her next visit, she came into my office and gave me a big hug! Then she proceeded to tell me that her PMS symptoms had completely disappeared! Somehow, the anterior pituitary gland supplement accomplished what all the other supplements could not.

The point is not that this, or any one substance or supplement, is the "answer" to any specific problem. The point is that all of the other nutrients weren't working for Helen—and the addition of a new one finally helped her.

The same may happen for you. You may find within these pages a supplement or two that will help make a critical difference in your life. We think that this kind of information about supplements is extremely valuable.

Most of the information in this book is backed up not only by clinical experience but also by stacks and stacks of impressive research published in prestigous medical journals. Some of it is a result of newly burgeoning research ambitiously, carefully, hopefully applied—and found effective. All of it is the result of people trying to find, and succeeding in finding, ways to help other people live healthier, stronger, happier, better lives.

2 Introducing the New Super Supplements

BEYOND VITAMINS, there is an exciting world of nutrients that could transform your life. These super supplements have solved persistent health problems in case after case. They may be able to raise the level of your health from fairly fit to super fit. All are worth knowing about. Some may prove to have tremendous personal value to you.

OUR FIRST STEP BEYOND VITAMINS: AMINO ACIDS

We all learned in grade school that amino acids are the building blocks of protein and that proteins are the building blocks of the body. There are 22 amino acids which combine in various ways to make the proteins that constitute the cells, tissues, organs, bones, nerves, and fluids that make up our body. Most of these amino acids can be synthesized in the body. But eight of them cannot, so they must be supplied in our diet. (The eight "essential" amino acids are isoleucine, leucine, lysine, methionine, phenylalanine, threonine, valine, and tryptophan.)

All of that is true—but it is also incomplete. We are learning that there is a lot more to the amino acid story.

Amino Acids' Vitaminlike Properties

We now know that many of the amino acids not only serve as structural components of proteins, but they also serve as factors in various crucial biochemical functions—just as the vitamins and minerals do. And, beyond vitamin- and mineral-type functions, the amino acids are also critical to the function of the brain.

We also know that although several amino acids can be made by the body, that doesn't necessarily mean the body is making enough for all of its needs. Theoretically, a diet that is adequate in high-quality protein should contain enough of all the essential amino acids to ensure synthesis of the others. Unfortunately, this isn't always the case. Apparently, many people do not get enough high-quality protein in their diets. And even if they do, various factors may prevent the body from synthesizing enough amino acids. In some cases the diet does not supply enough of other necessary raw materials, such as vitamins and minerals. In others, diseases or stresses of all kinds combine with genetic and metabolic factors to cause amino acid deficiencies.

These deficiencies behave much like vitamin deficiencies—they produce long-term, chronic symptoms that can progress into serious, acute problems. Amino acid deficiencies can impair the immune system, slow wound healing, and compromise our physical and mental performance—to name just a few of the consequences.

Some of the strongest evidence emerges from clinical experience: Supplements of individual and combined amino acids are helping to solve many stubborn health problems and improve people's levels of fitness, strength, and performance. For example, carnitine is a nonessential amino acid-like nutrient, which means that, theoretically, the body can manufacture all it needs. We know from clinical experience, however, that some people do have deficiencies of carnitine. Carnitine regulates the metabolism of fat in heart and skeletal muscle, so these deficiencies result in high blood and tissue levels of fat. When carnitine supplements are supplied, fat clearance from the body is improved. More fat is made available for energy, and blood and tissue levels drop.

Carnitine has other benefits, which we'll describe in later

chapters. But we want you to know that carnitine isn't the only amino acid that can have specific health benefits for you. In years to come, amino acids may equal vitamins and minerals as therapeutic agents in sickness, and preventive agents in health. In later chapters, we're going to explain how you can put amino acids to work for you right now.

ENZYMES:
YOU ARE WHAT YOU ABSORB

A popular maxim among nutrition-minded people is "you are what you eat." Today, with what we know about poor digestion, chronic diseases, aging, and our body's requirement for enzymes, that maxim might be more accurate if it stated: "You are what you absorb."

When we take our supplements or eat our meals, in our imaginations we may tally up how much of each nutrient the label says we're getting, and take for granted that we're actually absorbing and utilizing that amount. But we cannot make that assumption. We may be not be getting all the nutrients we think we are from either our supplements or our food, simply because we don't have enough of the enzymes we need for complete digestion and absorption of nutrients.

But incomplete digestion damages health in two ways: by inhibiting the absorption of necessary nutrients and by promoting the absorption of unnecessary and potentially harmful substances. In Chapter 10 we'll explain exactly how this seemingly contradictory situation arises—and how enzyme supplements can help correct it.

Enzymes Instead of Aspirin

Enzymes are useful for more than enhancing digestion. They can also help reduce inflammation caused by strains, sprains, and other minor injuries. In Chapter 7 we'll describe a nutrient combination that can be more effective than aspirin and other nonsteroidal drugs in reducing inflammation.

GLANDULAR SUPPLEMENTS: LIKE HEALS LIKE

To many people, the use of glandular supplements—which are concentrates of animal organs or glands—is the latest nutritional fad. Actually, however, glandular therapy is one of the oldest forms of medicine and glandular concentrates were among the very first supplements.

Glandular supplement therapy is relatively simple. If you know what organ or gland is ailing, or what gland controls the specific function you want to heal, you only need to find a supplement that contains the concentrate from that organ or gland, which has been extracted from animal tissue. Though several aspects of glandular therapy remain controversial, forms of glandular therapy are widely accepted among physicians not only in Europe, but also in the United States as well. We believe that the next few years will bring increasing scientific evidence of what glandular therapists have been saying for thousands of years: Like heals like.

When you get to Chapter 12 and the Beyond Vitamins Multisupplement Program, you will learn all about glandular therapy. Then, in later chapters, we will tell you how glandular supplements may help you boost your immunity, strengthen your response to stress, extend your youth, enhance the absorption of nutrients, and enhance your sex life.

BIOFLAVONOIDS: OUR PARTNERS IN GOOD HEALTH

Many nutritionally oriented physicians and researchers believe that bioflavonoids are among the hottest, most exciting supplements and that the immediate future holds even more promise. The excitement comes from recent discoveries showing a rapidly emerging role for bioflavonoids as supplements that not only prevent disease, but can also restore health.

Bioflavonoids are emerging as nutrients that can:

- Boost the immune system and help prevent and speed recovery from viral and bacterial infections
- Have a potent anti-inflammatory effect, without the side effects of steroids or aspirin
- Speed healing in athletic injuries and wounds
- Prevent cataracts and other eye disorders
- Prevent allergies and/or lessen their impact
- Help prevent cardiovascular disease and stroke
- Reduce menopausal symptoms
- Reduce excess bleeding
- Increase the efficiency of vitamins C and A
- Relieve pain from varicose veins, hemorrhoids, and leg swelling
- Stop bleeding, relieve pain, and speed healing of ulcers
- Relieve pain in arthritis
- Serve as antioxidants by scavenging free radicals
- Reduce bleeding and speed healing in periodontal disease
- Help detoxify carcinogenic chemicals

Vitamin P—The Potent Pretender

And yet, bioflavonoids are not vitamins. When they were first discovered more than 50 years ago, they were thought to be vitamins and were named "vitamin P." Nobody believes bioflavonoids are vitamins anymore, because they do not seem to be essential in quite the same way as vitamins and minerals are. When an essential vitamin or mineral is removed from the diet, specific deficiency symptoms eventually occur. This doesn't happen when bioflavonoids are experimentally removed from the diet. Bioflavonoids truly come into their own as supplements, as nutrients that are added to the diet to boost or regulate biological functions in a healthful way. They exert their effects in three ways: through the strengthening of the membrane and small blood vessel walls, by serving as antioxidants, and by regulating various key enzymes.

Bioflavonoids exist only in plants. Most of the yellow, red, and blue pigmentation in plants comes from the bioflavonoids. The principal sources of bioflavonoids are citrus fruits, particularly lemons and sweet oranges, but they are also derived from buckwheat, peppers, and other plants. Although there are over 800 naturally-occurring flavonoids, the three commonly used in supplements are rutin, quercetin, and hesperidin.

In later chapters we will explain the many ways in which you can make bioflavonoids your partners in good health.

ESSENTIAL OILS:
THE PRIMROSE PATH TO THE SEA
—AND BETTER HEALTH

Thanks to all the publicity surrounding heart disease, cholesterol, butter, margarine, and vegetable oils over the last two decades, most of us believe that the kind of oil we eat can make a difference in our state of health. That much is true, although the commercials trying to sell us margarine because of its supposed protective effects in cardiovascular disease are misleading.

Certain essential oils are better for us than others. And recent research has shown that some oils are not only essential in the same way that vitamins and minerals are, but that they can also have quite remarkable effects on health when they are included in the diet.

The Primrose Path . . .

The essential fatty acids (EFAs) have the same importance to the body as vitamins, in that they are required for certain metabolic reactions to take place, and because the body cannot manufacture them. In fact, they were originally identified as vitamin F. When the diet is deficient in EFAs, certain predictable symptoms develop, including hair loss, dry skin, painful joints, decline in liver function, fatigue, nervousness, sexual and fertility problems, and increased susceptibility to infections.

Until relatively recently, dietary oils were believed to be useful in only one way—to provide easily stored energy in the form of fat. Now we know that oils are required by the body for other biological functions, including the manufacturing of hormones and hormonelike chemicals that regulate a wide range of important biochemical reactions. These hormonelike chemicals are called prostaglandins, and they are especially important to regulating the immune system, the nervous system, and the cardiovascular system.

The Missing Step

There are several forms of prostaglandins, and the body requires a certain balance in order to remain healthy. Recent research has revealed, however, that in many people the biochemical steps that produce PG1 prostaglandins from linoleic acid are somehow blocked. Whether because of genetic or dietary factors, many people are lacking in one very important step—the conversion of linoleic acid to gamma-linolenic acid, or GLA. The enzyme responsible for the conversion is there, but may be diminished in activity because of aging, a high-saturated fat diet, or deficiencies of vitamin B_6, magnesium, or zinc. Fortunately, GLA can be obtained by eating certain oils, including that of the evening primrose plant and black currant seeds.

The Benefits of GLA

The rationale for supplementing the diet with GLA is to support the weakened or missing step in the production of PG1 prostaglandins. How important is the PG1 series? Very. PG1 prostaglandins play a pivotal role in:

- Reducing the tendency of blood to clot
- Widening blood vessels and preventing vessel spasms
- Reducing the severity and extent of heart damage during a heart attack
- Preventing and relieving angina pains
- Enhancing the energy-producing effects of insulin
- Healing ulcers caused by faulty circulation
- Supporting the immune system
- Reducing or preventing inflammation
- Relieving the pain and inflammation of arthritis
- Maintaining healthy, positive mood and mental functioning
- Supporting a healthy brain and nervous system

Therapeutically, GLA supplements, which boost the body's natural supply of PG1, have been used to:

- Relieve premenstrual syndrome
- Slightly improve the condition of people with multiple sclerosis
- Lower blood levels of cholesterol
- Lower high blood pressure
- Reduce the tendency of the blood to clot
- Improve circulation and relieve pain in people with intermittent claudication
- Restore healthy skin condition in people with eczema
- Relieve inflammation and pain in arthritis

- Reduce the toxic effects of alcohol
- Strengthen the immune system
- Reduce hyperactivity in children

To the Sea

GLA is only half of the essential oil story. The other half of the story began with the Eskimos. Some enterprising researchers investigated why the Eskimos, who eat a diet that is relatively high in animal fat, have so little heart disease. The scientists discovered that the Eskimos' diet included high levels of certain oils that were sharply reduced or absent in the diets of people with high risk of heart disease. These oils, EPA (eicosapentaenoic acid) and DHA (docosahexaenoic acid) are most commonly present in the oils of cold-water fish, such as cod, mackerel, sardines, herring, kippers, tuna, bonita, pilchard, butterfish, bluefish, and salmon.

Further research revealed that EPA and DHA stimulate the production of anti-inflammatory PG3 prostaglandins. We now know that EPA and DHA support health in many ways. They lower blood levels of LDL cholesterol, which is the harmful kind, and increase levels of HDL cholesterol, the helpful kind that is on its way out of the body. EPA and DHA also lower blood levels of other harmful fats, and reduce the tendency of the blood cells to clump together in dangerous clots. They serve to widen the blood vessels, thus reducing the possibility of a heart attack or stroke.

EPA and DHA are also potent anti-inflammatory agents. They compete with fatty acids that produce inflammatory prostaglandins and, instead, encourage the production of anti-inflammatory prostaglandins, such as PG1.

EPA and DHA have shown promise in preventing or treating many health problems that result from inflammation, including

- Food and environmental allergies
- Premenstrual syndrome
- Irritable bowel syndrome

- Psoriasis and eczema
- Arthritis
- Mood swings
- High blood pressure

Supplements of EPA and DHA are readily available; however, it is also possible to increase the amount of these oils in your diet by eating more cold-water fish.

One caution: Because EPA and DHA reduce the tendency of the blood to clot, they can worsen nosebleeds and perhaps cause easy bruising. Though the Eskimos are not prone to heart disease, they do tend to bruise easily.

THE OUTLAW VITAMIN: DIMETHYLGLYCINE

Dimethylglycine has enjoyed quite a checkered career as a supplemental nutrient. It has been called a vitamin, praised as a panacea, and outlawed by the FDA. More than 35 years ago, a substance was derived from apricot pits and other seeds, and named pangamic acid, or vitamin B_{15}. Subsequent research, particularly by the Russians, demonstrated some very extraordinary properties for this nutrient —although no one was able to prove that a lack of it in the diet produced a serious deficiency disease.

Russian research demonstrated that B_{15} supported the cardiovascular system, the liver, energy production and blood sugar metabolism, and boosted athletic performance. Some American physicians and nutritionists reported that B_{15} was of some benefit in treating autistic children.

We now know that the active ingredient in pangamic acid, and other forms of B_{15} such as calcium pangamate, is dimethylglycine, or DMG. DMG acts as a supportive intermediary in many biochemical functions involving vitamins, enzymes, hormones, neurotransmitters, RNA and DNA, and antibodies. DMG is not only a potent antioxidant and detoxifier, but it also improves the cell's use of oxygen and nutrients.

In later chapters we'll tell you how to put DMG to work for you to:

- Improve mental performance
- Boost strength and endurance
- Detoxify pollutants
- Protect the body against stress
- Strengthen the cardiovascular system
- Help the liver remove fat from the body
- Lower cholesterol levels
- Normalize blood sugar levels for more energy

ANCIENT NUTRIENTS ON THE CUTTING EDGE

Some of the newest supplements on the cutting edge of nutrition are among the oldest substances on earth. Some are relatively recent, whereas some have been with us all along, just hiding out in some foods that have always been old friends.

OCTACOSANOL—THE BONUS FROM WHEAT GERM OIL

Octacosanol sounds a lot more exotic than it really is. Although it sounds as if it might come from another planet, it's actually a concentrated nutrient derived from none other than an old-time health food favorite: wheat germ.

Nutrition scientists were on the trail of octacosanol way back in the 1930s, when they discovered that oils extracted from wheat germ had the ability to improve endurance and stamina. Later experiments revealed that the oil also reduced oxygen stress and quickened reaction time.

Researchers first assumed that the active ingredient in wheat germ oil was vitamin E, but comparative studies proved there was something else accounting for increased performance. Further analysis found that, in addition to vitamin E and essential fatty acids, wheat germ oil also contained several long-chain alcohol molecules. The performance-boosting effects of wheat germ oil were stimulated by these substances, one of which was octacosanol.

Later investigations have shown that these alcohols, of which octacosanol is highest in concentration, can have the following effects:

- Lower blood levels of cholesterol
- Improve energy storage in the muscles
- Improve endurance and stamina
- Quicken reflexes
- Improve performance at high altitudes
- Improve oxygen utilization
- Balance the metabolism under stress

Two things you should keep in mind when selecting octacosanol supplements: First, we recommend octacosanol derived from wheat germ oil only. Octacosanol synthesized from petroleum and other sources has not been tested, whereas the natural wheat germ oil variety has.

And second, the effects of octacosanol take upwards of three or more weeks to become noticeable.

GERMANIUM—EXCITING NEW SUPPLEMENT FROM JAPAN

Believe it or not, one of the most exciting and promising supplements is a rare mineral used in making transistors!

The Japanese, who have always had a knack for finding new ways to use transistors, have done most of the research on this nutrient. And they have found that it can:

- Improve mental alertness
- Lower high blood pressure
- Act as a potent anti-inflammatory
- Raise endorphin levels by inhibiting the enzyme that destroys these natural analgesics
- Rapidly stimulate interferon production to fight infections (especially viruses)
- Suppress tumors (in animal experiments)
- Boost the immune system

Germanium is not stored in the body, so 100 percent of what is taken in is excreted within two or three days. Thus there is no toxicity from excess storage, as there can be with other minerals. To date, the only nontoxic form of this mineral is the sesqui-oxide form.

Germanium is not quite as new as it may sound. Actually, garlic, ginseng, and other therapeutic herbs are quite high in this mineral. This fact makes for some vigorous speculation that some of the health-promoting powers of these herbs could be caused by germanium.

We suspect that the next "cutting edge" supplement on our list may also contain high concentrations of germanium.

CO-Q: THE LOST UBIQUITOUS NUTRIENT

Co-Enzyme Q, the newest supplement sensation from Japan, was actually isolated from heart cells more than 30 years ago. Originally called "Ubiquinone" (the ubiquitous quinone), it is a fat-soluble vitamin that is so essential to health that a 25 percent deficiency state can result in disease. Co-Q has been intensely studied for the past 20 years, mostly in the United States and Japan. Studies confirmed tremendous potential in:

- Stimulating the immune system
- Improving heart disease, angina, and congestive heart failure
- Reducing hypertension
- Healing periodontal disease
- Facilitating weight loss
- Boosting general energy and feeling of well-being
- Extending youth

Co-Q is present in many foods. It is richest in meat, especially organ meat; oily fish (the same that are high in EPA); and whole grains. There are ten types of Co-Q. Only $Co-Q_{10}$ is active in humans. Other forms must be converted to $Co-Q_{10}$ by the liver. $Co-Q_{10}$ blood levels have been found to decrease with aging, virus infections, in those with active heart disease, and suffering from malnutrition. The usual dose of $Co-Q_{10}$ is 20 mg. per day and it is apparently safe even in high doses.

MUCOPOLYSACCHARIDES— THE GLUE OF LIFE

Want to find out why oysters and mussels may really fulfill their role in folklore as aphrodisiacs? The answer may be in this difficult to pronounce—but very important —nutrient: mucopolysaccharides.

Mucopolysaccharides are natural substances that, together with collagen, form the glue that holds together all body tissues. Not only do they help account for the structural strength of tissues, but they also help regulate the transfer of nutrients, gases, and other substances through the cell walls. The effectiveness of the mucous membranes at keeping out invading organisms, the ability of the gut to absorb nutrients while keeping out larger proteins, and elasticity of the blood vessels and skin depend on the amount and quality of mucopolysaccharides present.

The body manufactures mucopolysaccharides, so it is unlikely that they will ever be designated as essential nutrients. There is evidence, however, that these substances not only decrease as we get older, but also deteriorate in quality. Furthermore, supplemental doses of mucopolysaccharides have shown to be beneficial in boosting health and improving symptoms in many diseases.

The mucopolysaccharides' major health-boosting properties stem from their ability to reduce inflammation, encourage healing and strengthen the tissues, and stimulate the immune system. They also reduce the tendency of the blood to clot, lower blood levels of cholesterol and other fats, promote growth and repair, and increase synthesis of nucleic acids DNA and RNA. Mucopolysaccharides are also very high in silicon, an essential mineral that promotes the strength of the connective tissue.

Supplements of mucopolysaccharides have been used to improve symptoms in arthritis, bursitis, respiratory disease, headaches (including migraine), ulcers, bedwetting, angina, and allergies.

Mucopolysaccharides feature prominently in the *Beyond Vitamins* Multisupplement—and, for reasons we'll explain later, in our Multisupplement program for a better sex life. This brand new supplement, it seems, may be the active ingredient in many ancient aphrodisiacs.

NOW YOU'RE READY TO JOURNEY BEYOND VITAMINS

Now that you've glanced at this road map of our Beyond Vitamins journey, we can explore how these nutrients— plus vitamins and minerals—build a better, more vigorous life. We're going to start, in the next few chapters, by building Beyond Vitamins Multisupplements and telling you how to use the supplement recommendations to get the fitness benefits you want most.

CHAPTER

3 The Basic Beyond Vitamins Supplement— Beginning to Answer the Questions: What to Take and How Much?

WHAT, EXACTLY, do we take and how much? These are the questions the Beyond Vitamins program is designed to answer. Starting with this chapter, you will learn how to build a customized supplement program that's all yours, designed to meet your needs.

There are two ways for you to use the information in this book—as a "program" and as a "bible." If you want guidance in designing a complete program using all or most of the Beyond Vitamins supplements, we will give you step-by-step instructions to help you do that. Using the book as a "bible," you don't have to take all of the supplements described in every chapter. If you want to choose individual Beyond Vitamins supplements that appeal to your needs, that's fine. You can use the dose range information in each chapter and in Chapter 15. We do, however, recommend that you first take the Basic Supplement as described in this chapter.

A PLACE TO BEGIN

This chapter will give you a jumping off place for your Beyond Vitamins program. We will give you baseline doses for the most basic vitamin and mineral supplements. Then, as you go through the rest of the book, you will be given information about specific supplements for your specific needs.

You may suspect that as you read through the chapters and add up the supplements, you will be overwhelmed by the accumulating doses! Don't be intimidated by all these lists of supplements. We will give you step-by-step instructions on how to design a simple, easy to follow personal program.

Please note, however, that you should NOT simply add up all the recommended doses. If, for example, you are a woman who is trying to boost immunity while fighting allergies, losing weight, and maximizing her mental and physical performance, adding up all the doses of all the potentially helpful supplements would create a mountain of pills!

It's a lot simpler than that. At the end of this book is your "Beyond Vitamins Workbook," which shows you how to design a total supplement program, combining supplements in a way that gets you the results you want efficiently and effectively.

Your Beyond Vitamins personal program Workbook in Chapter 15 contains a list of all the supplements described in this book. At the end of the chapter there are dose ranges for each nutrient mentioned in the chapter. If the specific benefits mentioned in that chapter are important to you, all you need to do is turn to the workbook, where you will find a list of all the Beyond Vitamins supplements, followed by columns that again give the dose ranges for all of the specific purpose chapters. As you go through the book, simply circle or mark the columns in the workbook that correspond to the specific nutritional purposes you desire.

When you've gone through the entire book, all you need to do to discover your dose range is look at your workbook and circle the lowest dose and the highest dose of each supplement, and then write it down in the space provided. That is your dose range for each supplement.

You will then have a list of all the supplements on your Beyond Vitamins personal supplement program. At that point, if you choose, you can simply start taking all of them at once. We recommend, however, that you follow our directions for beginning your personal supplement program a little at a time. We'll tell you where to start and how to add new supplements one at a time at regular intervals to allow you to take your steps beyond vitamins to a longer, healthier life.

And don't worry, we'll repeat all of our instructions again with the workbook.

BUILD YOUR FOUNDATION FIRST

A foundation supplement is a good idea in order to fill in the gaps that might be left by a specific supplement program. Also, you might be a person who is not losing weight, is perfectly satisfied with his or her performance, who never gets sick, and who doesn't have any allergies—and yet you want a baseline nutritional supplement to help keep things that way.

The Beyond Vitamins Basic Supplement

Vitamin A	10,000 I.U.
Carotene	20,000 I.U.
Thiamine	50 mg.
Riboflavin	50 mg.
Niacin	50 mg.
Pyridoxine	50 mg.
Pantothenic acid	100 mg.
Folate	400 mcg.
B_{12}	100 mcg.
Biotin	400 mcg.
Choline	250 mg.
Inositol	100 mg.
PABA	100 mg.

Vitamin C	1,000 mg.
Bioflavonoids	200 mg.
Vitamin D	200 I.U.
Vitamin E	200 I.U.
Calcium	500 mg.
Chromium	100 mcg.
Iodine	100 mcg.
Magnesium	250 mg.
Manganese	10 mg.
Molybdenum	50 mcg.
Potassium	100 mg.
Selenium	100 mcg.
Silicon	100 mg. (horsetail grass)
Zinc	30 mg.

BEYOND VITAMINS SUPPLEMENTS CAN MAKE A DIFFERENCE

I (M.R.) will give you an example of how Beyond Vitamins Supplements can make a difference.

Sally was one of my first patients. Though at 140 pounds she was about 10 pounds overweight for her 5 feet, 6 inch frame, she was still an attractive 29-year-old woman. A college graduate, Sally made program announcements and was responsible for scheduling at a San Francisco radio station. Her boyfriend was one of the station's DJs.

Sally's problem was that she could never depend on her energy supply. She complained of fatigue, aches and pains, headaches, and slight depression. Sally could function, but she had to push herself. Just about every morning she had to drag herself out of bed. Before her first cup of coffee, Sally felt grumpy, fuzzy-brained, and headachy. After her coffee she felt better and could begin her day. But at times throughout the day, she would feel fatigued, tense, irritable, and moody. She sometimes forgot names and phone numbers. At these times, she was temporarily relieved by eating a sweet snack or drinking a cup of coffee.

In my practice, I take the same medical history as any other physician, but I also spend additional time investigating a patient's diet in greater detail. In Sally's case, this important step revealed a lot.

Sally always drank her coffee with sugar. Her breakfast consisted of coffee with sugar and a sweet roll. Around mid-morning, Sally usually had another cup of coffee with sugar, and a muffin. Her lunch consisted of a tuna sandwich and more coffee. In the middle of the afternoon she had another cup of coffee. A typical dinner for her was pizza and soda pop.

By the time I got this far in her diet, Sally's fatigue was no mystery to me. But there was more. Sally spent a lot of time at her boyfriend's house. He lived with his father, who was a surgeon, and neither was much of a cook or a nutritionist. The refrigerator, Sally reported, was always filled with white bread, cakes, and other junk foods.

Sally's basic problem was too much sugar and coffee and not enough nourishing food. She got far too little protein in her diet. Whereas a woman of her size should have been getting about 45 grams of protein a day, she was getting only about 30. Added to this serious deficiency, Sally was addicted to caffeine. Her six cups of coffee each day amounted to almost 1,000 milligrams of caffeine. Her difficulty in waking up in the morning was simply withdrawal symptoms after going eight hours without caffeine. Then, throughout the day, Sally's fatigue and other mental symptoms were brought on not only by caffeine withdrawal but by the effects of all the sugar she was getting.

Finally, her boyfriend's eating habits only reinforced Sally's problems. She needed a big change. Fortunately, she was ready and willing to try new things.

I told Sally to stop all sweets and coffee "cold turkey" for three months. Some people can break their addictions better this way, while others need to change their habits a little at a time. In Sally's case, "cutting it cold" worked best. She was uncomfortable for about three weeks, but she could tell she was getting better. Her cravings for sugar and caffeine were slowly replaced with a healthy appetite for real food.

I also gave Sally a basic vitamin-mineral supplement because her blood tests indicated she was low in thiamine, pyridoxine, vitamin A, magnesium, and zinc. I also told her to eat more protein and more vegetables.

Sally steadily improved over the course of six to eight weeks. Her weight dropped 12 pounds and her energy levels and moods became steady and strong. I still hear from Sally occasionally. She continues to do well and never complains of fatigue. Sally has since added some new supplements to her personal program, including many of the nutrients described in this book.

A more recent case points out the progress we've made in using new supplements in helping people improve their health. Jane was a recent patient whose case is similar to Sally's. Jane was a 30-year-old assistant manager of a well-known nightclub in the North Beach district of San Francisco. Although Jane had a masters degree in marketing, she managed to cultivate a summer job as a hostess and part-time exotic dancer into a challenging and profitable career as a club manager.

Jane's major complaint was that she was afraid she was "losing it." She found herself either exhausted, angry, or depressed at times. Although her talent as a manager helped her get by, she worried that she would eventually damage her career.

Like Sally, Jane was too fond of sweets and coffee for her own good. Although she never touched the alcohol that was in abundance at her club, she drank seven or eight cups of coffee each day and indulged in Italian pastry from the bakery around the corner. Her only decent meal was a fish dinner at one of the district's renowned restaurants—but she only "indulged" herself that "luxury," as she called it, three or four times a week. The rest of the time she sent out for a sandwich.

With the more sophisticated blood and tissue tests available today, I found that Jane was deficient in just about every vitamin and mineral. Of course, I didn't need a test to tell me that. Jane's dietary report was all the information I needed.

Jane's tests also showed low levels of several amino acids. Here I was able to help her in a way that was unavailable for Sally ten years earlier. In addition to the vitamin and mineral supplements, I also gave Jane some amino acids. First, I told her to take a general amino acid supplement. Then, to help with her insomnia and anxiety, I gave her tryptophan. She took 1,000 mg. an hour before bed and 250 mg. between meals.

Of course, Jane also had to stop drinking coffee and eating sweets. To help her with this, I was able to give her glutamine (1,000 mg./day), an amino acid that helps reduce the craving for sweets. I gave her phenylalanine (1,000 mg./day) to help boost her moods during the withdrawal from caffeine. The mineral chromium helped balance her energy levels and further reduce her craving for sweets.

Jane reached the same steady state of energy and optimal performance that Sally did, but Jane did it faster and with less discomfort. Her withdrawal symptoms were not as severe and persistent as Sally's, thanks to the new supplements I was able to give her. These Beyond Vitamins Supplements can really make a difference!

PART II

Be Super Fit!

4 Nutrition Discoveries to Help You Thrive on Stress

REAL LIFE is impossible without stress. There is no way to completely avoid it. Yes, some ways of life are less stressful than others, but total deprivation from stress is impossible. If you somehow manage to isolate yourself completely from stress, that isolation itself will be stressful.

Besides, we like stress. We have an appetite for it, and if it's not appeased, we starve. Stress is wear and tear, but without it, there can be no growth and repair. We need a certain amount of stress to stimulate body and mind.

Unfortunately, life in the modern world brings with it stresses we can live without, such as anxiety and pollution of our air, water, and food supplies.

WHAT STRESS DOES TO US

Stress upsets our balance. All living things try their best to achieve and maintain balance. When the sun shines too brightly, they seek shade. When it gets too cold, they seek warmth. Not only do whole organisms try to maintain balance, but individual systems within organisms. In other words, there is an internal biological and chemical balance that the body wants to maintain, and there are some very sophisticated mechanisms set up to seek that balance. The scientific word for the body's balance is *homeostasis*.

When we're ticking along and the body is in balance, all of our biological systems operate in harmony. The right biochemicals are in the right places at the right times and everything hums along efficiently. Stress upsets that harmony. We'll give you an example from our personal experience.

One summer evening just before sunset, I (DB) was walking along beautiful Zuma beach here in southern California. The air was balmy and the Pacific Ocean was gentle and inviting. I stopped and watched the waves roll up the beach toward my feet. The water was too good to pass up. I stripped down to my bathing suit and ran into the ocean.

The exertion of running into the ocean and swimming out a few yards was a stress. It upset the nice balance my cardiovascular system had achieved in supplying oxygen and other nourishment to the cells of my body. In response to this stress, my body tried to restore balance. My heart beat faster and my breathing rate increased, so more blood, oxygen, and nourishment could be supplied to my cells, including my muscles, which were now doing more work. Because I'm in fairly good shape, balance was restored without a major upset. I reached a warm spot in the water about 15 yards out and just lay on my back and let the gentle waves rock me.

I rocked in the ocean for many minutes, wonderfully relaxed. There is actually no better way to achieve complete relaxation and isolation from stress than floating in warm water. Because the ocean was actually 20 degrees cooler than my body temperature, my heart pumped a little harder to maintain my body's temperature—again, maintaining balance. I was in such a blissful state that I just barely noticed the sun go down and the water turn from blue to black.

Suddenly, out of the corner of my eye, I caught sight of something flashing in and out of the water a few yards away. My attention was immediately riveted to the spot and . . . there it was again. It was a fin, slicing the black surface of the ocean between me and the shore.

Nothing drives home the concept of stress better than a fin in the water between you and the beach. In a split second, though nothing physically had happened to me, my body underwent enormous physiological adjustments. To put it mildly, my balance was upset.

My body froze, as if my blood had suddenly turned to ice. My muscles tensed. Rather than panicking, I was amazed to find that I was more alert. I could see better in the growing darkness. I could feel my heart pounding. Although I didn't reflect on it at the time, what was happening was this: My adrenal glands were squeezing out hormones to prepare my body for some form of gross physical action. My heart pumped harder, my blood pressure shot up, my blood vessels dilated to allow more blood to flow to my tense muscles. I felt the beginning of a cramp in my lower abdomen. I had a vision of myself pounding the attacker with my clenched fists.

Then I saw the fin again, this time about 20 yards further south than it had been. It was about the same distance from the beach as I was. But the fin seemed to be moving farther away, so I made my decision. I started swimming wildly for the beach. Only after several strokes did I realize that I was swimming with my fists clenched!

I didn't want to look for the fin, but I forced myself. It seemed closer. It was heading my way again—and there were two more fins near it! A new wave of terror streaked through me. I pushed myself even harder and started wondering when the water would get shallow enough for me to stand up and run. Strange, but despite all my frantic thrashing through the water, my mind was clear enough to consider how ridiculous it would seem to be chased by a fish through water shallow enough to run through!

Then my knee scraped against some small stones and my hand stroked through the shallow water right into the sand. I guess my mind had not allowed me to realize that, for the last few yards, I had been thrashing through water that was only a foot and a half deep.

I stood up, walked a few extra feet, and turned around.

The fin sliced the surface again. Then three others followed right behind. Then they came right up out of the water, slicing playful arcs. Dolphins.

I sat down on the beach and laughed. That was my conscious attempt to restore balance. I suppose the fact that I could laugh was a sign that my body and mind were prepared and able to get back the balance that had been so violently upset. Internally, my adrenal glands squeezed out some hormones that would signal the all clear. My blood pressure dropped, my heart and breathing rate slowed, my muscles relaxed somewhat.

I felt a shiver and started looking for my warm-ups. When I took a step I felt a pain in my knee. It was swollen and bruised. It hadn't bled much because part of my body's response to the "threat" was to increase the clotting ability of my blood. I hadn't felt cold or the pain of the bruise until now because my body's stress response had also somewhat anesthetized me with hormonelike substances called endorphins.

It wasn't easy to find my clothes in the dark. But I found them, put them on, and walked back to my car. I kept the heat on all the way home. By the time I arrived, got out of my damp clothes, showered, dressed, and ate some supper, I felt fine. Balance had been restored. My pulse was back to its resting rate of 60 beats per minute, and I was comfortably warm and well fed.

I had experienced some stress, my body had responded, and then it had restored balance.

Imagine this same kind of stress happening every day, several times a day. That may seem unlikely, but that's similar to what most of us experience. We may not have to face fins slicing through the ocean, but we face bad drivers and traffic jams, angry and insensitive bosses, friends and family with problems and bad tempers, the morning paper with its ominous headlines, the endless bills in the mail, the evening news that brings the world's problems into the living room . . .

Each one of these stresses upsets our balance and provokes a response similar to the one I experienced in the ocean. Each time the body does its best to restore balance. But when the stresses begin to accumulate, as they tend to do in modern life, the body has a tougher and tougher time restoring balance.

After a while, the body doesn't even try to restore the degree of balance it prefers. Instead, the body decides that it is always going to be upset and threatened—and it maintains a steady state that edges closer and closer to the state of alarm and readiness for gross physical action. Blood pressure remains high, the heartbeat continues to race, and breathing never returns to a relaxed state. The adrenal glands are continually taxed to provide hormones to regulate this state of alarm.

Keep in mind that in most of these cases, the circumstances that provoke the alarm response are not actual physical attacks, but because we are built the way we are, they are interpreted as attacks. I saw a fin in the water and my body did not wait to find out whether it was a shark or a dolphin. It was immediately interpreted as a threat. So it is with so many of the stresses of modern life.

ALL STRESS DRAINS OUR NUTRIENT RESERVES

But there are also stresses that are not a matter of interpretation, but which are actual physical attacks on the body's balance. The pollution of the air, water, and the food supply exposes us every day to real poisons that directly upset our biochemical balance.

All stress, whether it's pollution, an imagined threat, or even an activity such as exercise, which we do willingly in an effort to reduce our "alarm-response" stress, draws upon the body's biochemical resources in many ways.

1. Stress weakens us by upsetting our balance and using up our resources to restore balance.
2. Stress—of all kinds—creates toxic chemical by-prod-

ucts such as free radicals, which further damage living tissue. Toxic chemicals tax the body's detoxifying apparatus—that's fairly easy to understand. But even anti-stress activities such as jogging and bicycling create free radicals and inflammatory by-products, which will cause damage if they're not detoxified.

The liver is the major detoxifier in the body. Various enzymes and other biochemicals do the detoxifying work there. But these biochemicals have to come from somewhere, don't they? They come from our food. Rather, we should say that, *ideally*, they come from our food. If they're not supplied in the diet, then they're not supplied at all, and the toxins are allowed to weaken us even more.

3. Stress, by weakening us and drawing down our resources, leaves us more vulnerable to such degenerative diseases as diabetes, arthritis, cancer, and heart disease.

4. Stress makes us older, mainly by using up our resources. Stress puts pressure on all our biological machinery that works to maintain the balance in our favor. To some extent, that machinery needs the stimulation—as long as we are providing it with the nutrients it needs. If we don't, then our reserves of these vital nutrients are drained and all biological functions will suffer the loss. Stress is a catalyst, it activates and amplifies the effects of all the other causes of disease and aging (see Chapter 6), and accelerates the use and loss of nutrients.

THE ACCUMULATION OF TOXINS TAKES ITS TOLL

In addition to the poisonous chemicals that enter the body through our air, food, and water, the body creates toxins of its own, as necessary by-products of metabolic functions. Ideally, the body is able to cleanse itself and neutralize these toxins, but as we get older and live through more stress, these toxins begin to accumulate. As our ability to detoxify them deteriorates, the damage wrought by these toxins increases. They interfere with the cells' ability to reproduce, as well as their ability to function in a normal, healthy fashion.

Stress increases the body's accumulation of toxic by-products. When we're under a lot of stress, metabolic waste products are created at a faster rate and the body's ability to detoxify them and remove them can be severely taxed.

STRESS CREATES FREE RADICALS

Free radicals are the biochemical vandals that scientists believe do most of the actual dirty work of stress, many diseases, and aging. They damage the blood vessels, oxidize fatty acids, cross-link molecules, damage our DNA and RNA, aid in the deterioration of the immune system and the damage done by autoimmune aging, contribute to the decline in our neurotransmitters, and either help trigger or actually execute the aging wrought by the mysterious "aging clock."

A free radical is a molecule that is incomplete—and "angry" about being only a fragment. The restless fragment is anxious to collide with another molecule so it can combine and achieve some form of chemical balance. That balance is achieved at the expense of the molecule that becomes the free radical's target, which is likely to be damaged. In some cases, free radicals do not directly damage the molecules, but instead create new molecules that hamper cellular functions or have direct toxic effects. Free radicals can also pull together molecules that aren't normally joined, in a "cross-link" that disrupts the molecule's original function. (More about cross-linking in the next chapter).

Free radicals are not totally villainous. Not only are they responsible for the dirty work of aging, but also for a lot of the body's legitimate dirty work. The body produces a small amount of free radicals for use by the immune system, for example, to kill bacteria, viruses, and cancer cells. Free radicals are also put to good use in the body's synthesis of vitamin D. To keep them under control, the body also manufactures two potent antioxidant enzymes: glutathione peroxidase and superoxide dismutase.

Sometimes the body's own free radicals get loose and cause trouble. Free radicals are generated constantly as the cells burn sugar to produce energy. Stress creates free radicals, by increasing the amounts of noradrenaline in the blood. Radiation from x-ray machines, nuclear power plant accidents, TV sets, microwave ovens, sunlight, and cosmic rays creates free radicals, as does air pollution, cigarette smoke, ozone, and other toxic materials in the environment. One of the major sources of free radicals is the oxidation of lipids, or fatty acids, in the body. Not only do fatty acids circulate in the blood, they also make up important structural parts of every cell.

Free radicals and oils, or fatty acids, are dangerous because the oxidation of the oils creates still more free radicals . . . which oxidize more fatty acids and create more free radicals . . . on and on.

To understand just how important free radicals are, consider the fact that we don't know of a part of the body that is not damaged by free radicals, just as we do not know of a disease that does not in some way make use of free radicals.

ANTISTRESS NUTRIENTS

Nutrients that help us respond to and resist the damaging effects of stress include those that will help us detoxify pollutants and toxic by-products of stress, free radical scavengers and antioxidants, and also nutrients known to strengthen the body's resources against stress. Finally, some antistress nutrients may help by actually relaxing us, thus decreasing the severity of the alarm response.

The combined effects of stress can take many forms, many of them hidden. Let us give you an example.

Hillary was a thirty-two-year-old artist. I (MR) knew she was creative the moment she walked into my office. Her clothes were a carnival of bright colors. Unfortunately, her mood was not as festive as her clothes. Hillary made her living as an artist, but like many artists, she had her financial ups and downs. Now, Hillary complained that the ups and downs were starting to get to her. Whereas before she had always handled the insecurity by plunging into her work with renewed vigor, now she found that energy was more elusive than ever before.

Her work was suffering. She was often too tense to even mix her paints, let alone create a picture. Her palms would sweat, her heart would race. She was having trouble sleeping, and was waking up in the middle of the night—terrified.

For two years, Hillary had tried psychotherapy, which had relieved her anxiety only slightly. She complained that it seemed to dredge up more problems than it solved. She had also taken prescribed tranquilizers, but she had disliked their side effects.

I could find no serious shortcomings in Hillary's diet. And her tests did not indicate any abnormalities. I came to the conclusion that she was suffering from anxiety caused by the unusually stressful insecurity of her career. I have seen attorneys and stockbrokers suffer the same symptoms.

In Hillary's case, I suggested that she take a basic multi-supplement, plus many of the antistress nutrients described in this chapter. In particular, I told Hillary to take 1,000 mg. of tryptophan one hour before she went to bed, and then 250 mg. three times during the day, always on an empty stomach. Hillary reported that she slept better almost immediately, and that her anxiety was relieved. She could work again!

I further advised Hillary that she should not take tryptophan every night, but only when she anticipated an especially anxious period in her life. This program has worked well for her. She reports that she uses tryptophan about five or six days and nights each month and that her career is flourishing. In Hillary's case, stress was weakening her and visibly preventing her from enjoying the fruits of her natural talents. Now she is able to strengthen herself against the stress caused by the insecurity of her chosen field.

We all have insecurities and anxieties, whether we're artists, accountants, parents, or princes.

THE BASIC ANTISTRESS B VITAMINS

The B vitamins have always been known as antistress nutrients. Many antistress supplement formulas contain little more than the B vitamins. Although we believe the B vitamins are a good place to begin fighting stress, a complete antistress program goes beyond the Bs—and beyond vitamins.

Because of their importance to our energy supply and the health of the adrenal glands, the B vitamins help us resist stress. Thiamine, riboflavin, and pyridoxine are vital to energy metabolism and, therefore, to resisting stress. Pyridoxine also helps the liver detoxify poisonous chemicals and metabolic by-products. Through its support of the adrenal glands pantothenic acid is a crucial anti-stress nutrient.

The B vitamins also help us deal with the effects of the alarm response. Niacin can help reduce anxiety, depression, insomnia, apprehensiveness, and fatigue—as well as lower cholesterol and dilate the blood vessels to increase circulation. Many of the other B vitamins also help the nervous system handle the stresses and strains of modern life.

The B vitamins also came to be known as antistress nutrients because they are often the first deficiencies to develop during periods of stress. Water-soluble nutrients, such as the B vitamins, vitamin C, and all of the minerals, are generally excreted at a faster rate during periods of stress. Because the B vitamins (and vitamin C) are not stored to any great extent, deficiencies can develop rather quickly. Most mineral deficiencies tend to develop over longer periods of time, because many minerals are, to some extent, stored in the bones and tissues.

NUTRIENTS THAT ROUND UP FREE RADICALS

Though the B vitamins are the time-honored antistress nutrients, recent research has shown us that the key to resisting stress lies in neutralizing free radicals and preventing oxidation. An antioxidant molecule serves its function by sacrificing itself for oxidation, thus protecting vulnerable tissues. The nutrients that help protect us against free radicals are the antioxidants. Vitamin C is the principal water-soluble antioxidant. It helps protect the entire body, including the brain and nervous system, from free radical damage. Vitamin C also indirectly helps fight oxidation in the fatty layers of the cells, by converting oxidized vitamin E back to its antioxidant form.

Vitamin E is the major fat-soluble antioxidant. It protects the fatty acids within the cells, including those in the blood, from free radicals. Vitamin E is our principal protector against ozone, the common air pollutant, which damages the lungs and other tissues through oxidation. We now know that as ozone levels in the air rise, tissue stores of vitamin E drop—even in people receiving "adequate," or RDA-type amounts in their diets.

Thanks to recent research, we now know that beta-carotene is also a major antioxidant nutrient, on a par with vitamin E, and very similar to vitamin E in that it protects the fatty layers of the cells from free radicals.

Selenium is the principal mineral antioxidant and free

radical deactivator. Selenium is a cofactor in glutathione peroxidase, the body's own free radical controller. Other cofactors include zinc, manganese, and copper. Selenium and vitamin E potentiate each other's effectiveness against free radicals.

Another important antioxidant is the peptide (a substance similar to an amino acid) glutathione. Glutathione is produced by the combination of the amino acids glutamic acid, cysteine, and glycine. One way in which glutathione serves as an antioxidant is by converting oxidized vitamin C back to a form in which it can go off and once again serve as an antioxidant. Glutathione peroxidase, one of the major antioxidants manufactured by the body itself, requires the presence of glutathione and selenium.

Zinc is also a key antistress, antioxidant nutrient. Zinc serves as an antioxidant by stimulating the activity of superoxide dismutase, which is the second antioxidant produced by the body. We want you to understand how incredibly important zinc is to our resistance to stress. Tests have shown that whenever we're subjected to stress, zinc is mobilized and blood levels rise considerably. We believe that zinc is, like adrenal hormones, part of the body's front line anti-inflammatory response to stress. The rise in blood levels and the three- to five-fold increase in the excretion of zinc during stress indicate that the body wants to increase the amount of zinc available to tissues— a sure sign that it's vital.

NUTRIENTS THAT HELP DETOXIFY POLLUTANTS

Any nutrients that support the liver will help the body detoxify itself. Principal liver-supporting and detoxifying nutrients include vitamin A, the B vitamins, and vitamin C. Vitamin C helps protect the body against the harmful effects of alcohol, cadmium, lead, nitrates (which are in processed foods), vanadium, PCBs, pesticides, and chlorine in drinking water. Add a pinch of ascorbic acid to chlorinated water and you will instantly neutralize the chlorine taste.

Several minerals help to detoxify poisonous heavy metals that pollute our air, water, and food supply. The principal detoxifying minerals are calcium, selenium, and zinc.

The amino acid cysteine is also a major detoxifier. It is the body's main source of sulfur and it helps detoxify mercury, silver, cobalt, cyanide, and acetaldehyde (from cigarettes and alcohol).

NUTRIENTS TO REDUCE BLOOD FATS

During periods of stress, levels of blood fats such as cholesterol and triglycerides tend to rise. Lipotropic substances, such as methionine, DMG, and choline, and other nutrients known to aid the liver and promote fat burning, such as vitamin A, vitamin C, the B vitamins, carnitine, taurine, and liver substance will help the liver keep blood fats to a minimum.

NUTRIENTS TO TURN OFF
THE BODY'S ALARM

Detoxifying the poisons and poisonous by-products of stress is only half the battle. The other half consists of reducing the constant state of alarm that stress provokes. As we already mentioned, the B vitamins help by supporting the nervous system and the adrenal glands, both of which are essential to turning off the alarm response and promoting relaxation. Vitamin C strengthens the adrenal glands, which not only help turn on the alarm response, but also are required to turn it off.

The minerals calcium, potassium, and magnesium will help reduce the effects of stress primarily by lowering blood pressure and allowing the muscles to relax. Magnesium, in particular, lowers blood pressure by relaxing the blood vessels and the vascular smooth muscle cells.

The amino acids tyrosine and phenylalanine are helpful in turning off the alarm response. Phenylalanine lowers stress-induced high blood pressure, lowers stress-induced blood fats and blood sugar, and reduces constriction of the bronchial tubes. Phenylalanine also helps relieve depression.

Tyrosine carries out many of the same tasks as phenylalanine, perhaps because phenylalanine is converted by the body into tyrosine. Tyrosine helps raise antistress hormones, which lower the alarm response. It also lowers high blood pressure. Actually, it normalizes blood pressure: In cases of shock, where blood pressure falls to abnormally low levels, tyrosine is used to raise the blood pressure.

ANTISTRESS, ANTI-INFLAMMATORY NUTRIENTS

Stress can induce a state of generalized inflammation over the entire body, or in specific parts of the body. High blood pressure is part of this generalized inflammation. Muscle soreness and fatigue, and joint stiffness are also symptoms of inflammation. To the extent that certain nutrients can reduce inflammation, they can also be thought of as antistress nutrients.

The B vitamins, particularly B_6, niacin, and folic acid help reduce inflammation and keep the blood vessels from constricting.

Anti-inflammatory nutrients, such as bioflavonoids, the enzyme bromelain, and essential fatty acids from fish oil should also help. Fish oils, you will remember, contain fatty acids EPA and DHA, which were found to be the active ingredients that greatly reduce the risk of cardiovascular disease. They not only lower blood levels of dangerous fats such as cholesterol, but they also lower blood pressure. Fish oils containing EPA and DHA have also been shown to be beneficial in reducing inflammation and relieving arthritis symptoms.

Mucopolysaccharides will not only help reduce inflammation, but will also help maintain the strength and elasticity of the blood vessels.

Stress raises blood sugar and stimulates high levels of insulin secretion, which, in itself, can stress the blood vessels and tissues. To help keep blood sugar balanced and reduce the need for high blood levels of insulin, glucose-tolerance-factor chromium should be used. Chromium is a cofactor for insulin, and increases the efficiency of the hormone, thus making less of it necessary to control blood sugar.

OTHER ANTISTRESS NUTRIENTS

DMG is also an effective antistress nutrient. By boosting energy levels and helping to detoxify pollutants, DMG helps us battle stress. DMG can improve endurance, strength, and stamina under physical and mental stress. It also boosts adrenal function.

The amino acid arginine prevents stress-induced weakening of the immune system (more about arginine and the immune system in the next chapter).

The principal antistress glandular supplement is adrenal substance. The adrenal glands are responsible for orchestrating the body's response to stress. That means not only do these glands help tune up and rouse the body's "stress musicians" to action, but they also modulate them and tell them when to put their instruments away and go home. When the adrenals become overtaxed, the body can become exhausted by becoming stuck in a perpetual state of alarm.

Any regenerative help from adrenal glandular substance may come in handy.

The Beyond Vitamins Multisupplement to Resist Stress

For additional information on how to design your personal Beyond Vitamins Program, see Chapter 15.

VITAMINS

Vitamin A	10,000 I.U.
Carotene	25,000 I.U.
Thiamine	50 mg.
Riboflavin	50 mg.
Niacin	50–200 mg.
Pyridoxine	50 mg.
Pantothenic acid	100–1,000 mg.
Folate	400 mcg.
B_{12}	100 mcg.
Biotin	400 mcg.
Choline	250 mg.
Inositol	100 mg.
PABA	100 mg.
Vitamin C	1000–10,000 mg.
Bioflavonoids	200–1,000 mg.
Vitamin E	200–400 I.U.

MINERALS

Calcium	500–1000 mg.
Chromium	200 mcg.
Magnesium	200–500 mg.
Potassium	200 mg.
Selenium	100–200 mcg.
Zinc	50 mg.

AMINO ACIDS

Arginine	100 mg.
Carnitine	100 mg.
Methionine	100 mg.
Cystine	100 mg.
Glutathione	200–500 mg.

Glycine	100 mg.
Glutamic Acid	100 mg.
Cysteine	100 mg.
Taurine	100 mg.
Tyrosine	100–500 mg.
or Phenylalanine	200–500 mg.

OTHERS
EPA	500–1,000 mg.
GLA	40 mg.
Mucopolysaccharides	200 mg.
DMG	100–200 mg.

ENZYMES
Bromelain	100–500 mg.

GLANDULARS
Adrenal	50 mg.
Liver	50–500 mg.

CHAPTER

5 Boost Your Immunity Beyond Vitamins

IT'S A dangerous world, there's no question about it. And it doesn't seem to be getting any less dangerous, either. As this chapter is being written, the entire medical world has been mobilizing for a war against one of the most insidious and deadly diseases ever known—AIDS, or, Acquired Immune Deficiency Syndrome.

While scientists wrestle with the research and try to come up with a new medical miracle to combat this dread disease, most of us watch the ever-escalating statistics and wonder what we can do to protect ourselves and our loved ones. At this point, we can do two things:

1. Hope and pray that the research will yield some answers and some effective drugs as soon as possible.
2. Apply what we know about the prevention of other viral diseases and general support of the immune system to our personal health programs.

It's number 2 that this chapter is going to address. We don't want to mislead anyone into thinking that we believe we have the cure for AIDS. By now we should all know that AIDS (and other serious diseases) are much too complicated to be solved with simple measures.

BOOST YOUR IMMUNE STRENGTH ALL YOU CAN

Our aim is to present Beyond Vitamins supplements that can boost the effectiveness of your immune system and strengthen it against many diseases and toxins, not just AIDS. After all, we believe that although most people are concerned about AIDS, the great majority of us face more real day-to-day threats from more common diseases, such as flu, herpes, the common cold, cancer, and other diseases that rely on or cause a weakened immune system. As a matter of fact, even if AIDS did not exist, strengthening our immune system would still be a major priority. Many of the diseases of the twentieth century are the result of a weakened immune system.

Candida—A Twentieth-Century Disease

Candida (Albicans) is a yeast organism that has learned how to live in humans. Most of us carry the organism without symptoms, as is the case with other yeasts. But many people—particularly women—suffer a wide range of symptoms because of this organism's particular adaptation to twentieth-century conditions. The yeast thrives on sugar, which, unfortunately, is a dietary mainstay in today's world. The widespread use of antibiotics has aided the spread of *Candida* by killing off beneficial bacteria that control the disease-producing organisms. The yeast also appears to have an affinity for female hormones. Birth control pills are a boon to *Candida*.

Furthermore, not only does the yeast take advantage of a weak immune system, but it also seems to have the ability to further weaken the immune system.

Candida causes inflammations in the stomach and digestive tract, bladder, and vagina. Bladder infections, vaginal discharges, diarrhea, indigestion, fatigue, depression, malaise, skin rashes, and susceptibility to other infections may result. *Candida* itself prefers warm, moist surfaces and doesn't survive on the skin. Skin problems are caused by cousin yeasts that may take hold.

In some people, the original infection combines with an allergy to yeast, in which case the symptoms can be debilitating. This hypersensitivity can be treated in much the same way that an inhalant allergy is treated, by administering a desensitization shot.

To stimulate the immune system to fight off the *Candida* infection itself, in addition to the measures described in this chapter, it's best to remove all sugar, sweets, alcohol, and overripe fruits (which contain mold as well as high levels of sugar) from the diet, because the *Candida* organism thrives on sugar. Also a good idea: supplements of garlic, which directly kill the yeast, and acidophilus bacteria, which restore beneficial bacteria in the gut.

EBV—THE SINISTER ENERGY THIEF

Another twentieth-century disease is the Epstein-Barr virus (EBV) infection. Although the virus has been around for millions of years, during recent years the Epstein-Barr virus has been revealed to be responsible for a lot of illness that was misdiagnosed or undiagnosed. A lot of people—perhaps hundreds of thousands—complained to their doctors that waves of exhaustion, depression, aches, and pains came over them without warning and rendered them useless for work or play. Some people experience this one or two days a month, some have it almost every day and can't function at all.

Doctors couldn't find anything "wrong" with these people—their standard lab tests showed nothing abnormal. So one of three diagnoses was made: either the patient was malingering, overstressed, or in need of a psychiatrist. Many of the victims of EBV also became the victims of the fact that the doctors couldn't figure out what was wrong with them. Without a formal diagnosis, social service agencies, workmen's compensation, and employers were refusing to assist people who were desperately ill. As far as these agencies were concerned, there was nothing wrong with them!

Then we learned that their problems were being caused by the Epstein-Barr virus, which is the same virus that causes mononucleosis. Like many other viral infections, the EBV "hides" in the body for many years and emerges to produce symptoms at opportune times, such as when stress or other factors weaken the immune system.

We don't know how to eradicate this disease. But we do know that although the EBV is a fairly common virus, it doesn't make everyone sick. Until something better comes along, our best plan is to stimulate the immune system all we can. In addition, mononuclcosis should be taken seriously, instead of viewed with the casual attitude most people have toward it. Many people who have had mono report that they've never regained their full strength and general good health. The strength of the immune system before, during, and after the initial infection must play a key role in determining what kind of foothold the virus will take in the body.

We want to apply what we know about fortifying the immune system against these twentieth-century diseases. First, let's take a look at our immune system and how it works, so we can better appreciate why certain supplements can help boost our defenses.

OUR PERSONAL IMMUNE FORCES

Our immune system is our personal armed forces. And just as our country has an army, an air force, a navy, a coast guard, and marines, the immune system also has different branches of service. Because all kinds of enemies threaten the body—bacteria, viruses, fungi, tumors, foreign proteins, toxic materials—each branch has its own specialty and its own battle strategies.

The branches of our immune force include the cellular immune force, which includes the various cells that go out to battle invaders; the humoral force, which consists of the various immune chemicals that circulate in the body; and, finally, the various immune system organs and glands themselves.

The organs and glands of the immune system include the thymus gland, whose responsibility it is to "teach" lymphocytes what enemies to attack; the bone marrow, where lymphocytes are manufactured; and the spleen, where lymphocytes are stored.

The cellular immune force includes the various white blood cells. Of these, the lymphocytes are the primary attack group, and the phagocytes are the powerful second wave. At any given time, more than a trillion lymphocytes should be circulating in the body or on guard in the lymphatic system. These lymphocytes actually are a twin force, consisting of B cells and T cells.

T CELLS ARE THE MINUTEMEN OF THE IMMUNE SYSTEM

The T cells are the front line sentries. It's their job to sound the alarm, call the other defending forces to the battle, and mount the first attack. The T cells attack by manufacturing chemicals that kill bacteria, viruses, and fungi.

How do the T cells know what to attack? They are "taught" by the thymus gland or, more precisely, by thymosin, the hormone secreted by the thymus gland. The T cells are instructed how to distinguish between "not self" and "self," between foreign proteins and the body's own proteins.

THE SECOND WAVE

The second wave attack is mounted by the phagocytes, or macrophages, which are white blood cells that actually devour the invading proteins. Phagocytes use free radicals to destroy the invaders. Because free radicals are so promiscuously toxic, the phagocytes must also carry adequate antioxidants to protect themselves.

The immune system has more in its armory. Remember the B cells? The B cells, which are "matured" in the lymph nodes and spleen, become plasma cells that produce antibodies. Antibodies are vital—and unique—because they give the immune system a memory. Once the plasma cells have produced antibodies against a specific invader, they never forget an unfriendly face. They continue to produce antibodies—and then go into high gear if the invader attacks again. Each time the invader returns, it is fought off with increasing efficiency, often without noticeable symptoms.

The existence of antibodies makes immunization possible and explains why we get diseases like chicken pox and measles only once. We can also test to learn whether we have been exposed to a certain disease by checking to see whether the immune system has produced antibodies against it.

Circulating antibodies patrol the blood, and secretory antibodies patrol the saliva and the mucosal fluids of the respiratory, gastrointestinal, and genitourinary tracts—often the first places invading organisms attack. We know that extreme stress and a deficiency of vitamin A can lower our production of secretory antibodies.

Histamines and interferon are two principal chemicals used by the immune system. Histamine produces inflammation, which may be good for fighting off invaders, but not so good when the immune system mistakes pollen, hair from a friend's cat, or one of our favorite foods for a dangerous invader. Interferon is very important to our defense against cancer and viruses.

THE AGING OF OUR IMMUNE SYSTEM

If our immune system remained as powerful as it was when we were 10 years old, we'd probably live more than 100 years. Unfortunately, once we pass adolescence, the immune system starts to decline slowly. The principal reason for this decline is the shrinking of the thymus gland. As the gland shrinks, it produces less thymosin, the hormone that trains T cells. When the T cells aren't trained as completely as they could be, our immune system weakens.

The pituitary gland secretes a hormone, called growth hormone, which stimulates and maintains the thymus gland. But the pituitary gland also changes as we grow out of our teens, and produces less growth hormone. The aging pituitary may also secrete a hormone that purposely blocks the release of thymosin.

Clearly, if we want to maintain our immune strength, we need to take definite steps to bolster the immune system.

Here's an example: Merrill was a thirty-six-year-old airline pilot who was on the verge of being grounded by persistent, recurring respiratory infections. Hardly a month went by that he didn't spend at least three days in bed with the flu and several days nursing a cold. Because he was sick so often, Merrill was afraid that he would have to leave his senior position and fly only part-time. Most cold medications contain sedatives, so when he was sick, he had to stay home.

Merrill was already taking a high-quality stress supplement, but I (MR) explained to him that he needed some extra support for his immune system. I advised him to add 25,000 I.U. of vitamin A, 25,000 I.U. of carotene, 400 I.U. of vitamin E, 200 mcg. of selenium, 100 mg. of zinc, and 5,000 mg. of vitamin C to his daily program. On days when he felt a cold coming on, I told him he might add another 5,000 mg. of vitamin C. I also suggested that he take 200 mg. of glutathione, 1,000 mg. of ornithine, and 250 mg. of taurine every day.

Merrill reported back a month later. He said it was the first month in more than three years in which he hadn't lost a day of work because of the flu or a bad cold. He did have two colds during the month, but they were not serious. His Beyond Vitamins Supplement Program was beginning to make a difference in his life.

Over the next few months, Merrill continued to make progress. When he felt a cold coming on, he would increase his vitamin C and, more often than not, he was able to fight off the infection. When he went four months without as much as a cold, we agreed that his immune system was once again doing its job and that he could cut his supplements in half. Merrill still doubles his supplements when he feels threatened by an infection, but he hasn't lost a day of work in over a year.

NUTRITIONAL IMMUNITY FACTORS

The first and foremost nutritional component of a powerful immune system is protein. Yes, protein. Acquired immune deficiency caused by protein-energy deficiency is much more common than that caused by the AIDS virus. The immune system carries on a relatively rapid turnover of cells, so there must be adequate protein available for the timely production of new immune components. T cells, secretory antibodies (the first line of the immune system), the phagocytes, the integrity of the mucosal surfaces, and interferon production are all reduced in Protein-Energy Malnutrition (PEM).

Don't assume that protein-energy malnutrition is a factor only in undeveloped countries, for it exists in the United States as well. In many acute care hospitals, researchers have found more than 15 percent of the patients suffering from PEM serious enough to compromise the immune system. Were these patients admitted to the hospital with malnutrition? Not always. Many of them became malnourished while in the hospital. Because AIDS can be transmitted through blood transfusions, and because blood transfusions are generally administered to hospital patients after some stressful, immunity-damping trauma such as surgery or injury, adding malnutrition only heightens the danger.

How do you know how much protein is right for you? As with all nutrients, we each have our own individual requirements. Women, who generally have lower concentrations of muscle and higher concentrations of fat than men do, can require less protein. A good general guideline for protein intake can be arrived at in the following way: First find your weight in kilograms. (If your bathroom scale is not calibrated in kilograms, simply divide your weight in pounds by 2.2.) Then, if you're a man, multiply your weight in kilograms by .7. If you're a woman, multiply your weight in kilograms by .6. The number you get is your approximate daily protein requirement in grams of protein. Now you know how much protein you need each day to maintain a strong immune system.

Protein and calorie deficiencies aren't the only factors in PEM immune suppression. Nutritional cofactors that support protein metabolism and synthesis, including zinc, pyridoxine, and folic acid, are also important factors. As a matter of fact, zinc may be the key factor in PEM immune suppression. In some cases, weakening of the immune system during PEM can be traced to zinc deficiency, and raising zinc levels—even without restoring adequate protein—can boost immune strength to normal levels.

COMMON IMMUNE SABOTEURS

You should also be aware of some common substances and supplements that can weaken the immune system. Women, for example, should be aware of two important facts: First, progesterone, which is used in birth control pills and as a treatment for premenstrual syndrome, is a steroid hormone and, like all steroid hormones, may suppress the immune system. (Vitamin D, which also qualifies as a steroid hormone, can also suppress the immune system when taken in excess amounts. Unless your physician has specifically recommended vitamin D supplements, you should not take more than is normally present in a multivitamin formula.)

Second, iron (although required for adequate immune strength) in excess amounts can also result in reduced immunity to bacterial infections, particularly in situations where protein-energy nutrition is inadequate—as it might be during a "crash" diet. The excess iron does not specifically damage the immune system—it actually strengthens the invading bacteria. Therefore women should be careful not to take excessive supplements of iron, especially when they feel threatened by a bacterial infection. There is no evidence that men routinely require daily iron supplements.

A very common food item is also capable of weakening our body's defenses. A high intake of polyunsaturated fatty acids can produce a profound suppression of the immune system, including accelerated deterioration of the thymus gland. It is not known what precise level of polyunsaturated fatty acids in the human diet will produce immunosuppression. Because of their immunity-weakening effects plus their ability to increase the body's load of free radicals, excessive amounts of polyunsaturated oils increase our risk of cancer and cardiovascular disease.

However, a deficiency of essential fatty acids (which are

supplied by vegetable oils) also produces immune depression. Clearly, we need some unsaturated oils in our diets. Polyunsaturated oils, however, are not the best sources, when their instability and their immune suppressing abilities are taken into account. Olive oil and peanut oil, which are monounsaturated rather than polyunsaturated, supply some essential fatty acids, but are more stable and less likely to weaken the immune system.

THE BEYOND VITAMINS
IMMUNITY BOOSTERS

Several nutrients and supplements are especially effective because they help stimulate the immune system to work more efficiently and accurately. We'll start with the vitamins and minerals, because many people don't know how these old standby supplements can boost the strength of the immune system.

Vitamin A—Immune Stimulant Extraordinaire

Vitamin A keeps the mucous membranes in top working order. Maybe you never stopped to think about your mucous membranes, but they are your first line of defense against any unwanted organism or substance that tries to enter the vulnerable interior of your body.

Vitamin A promotes the production of lysozymes (anti-infectious agents) in tears, saliva, and sweat and also directly strengthens the immune system by stimulating the all-important thymus gland.

Megadoses of vitamin A have been shown to reverse the immunity-dampening effect of surgery. This immuno-suppression normally lasts up to three or four weeks. However, megadoses of vitamin A (300,000 IU/day) for one week after extensive surgery not only blocked the expected immunosuppression but actually increased immune strength in the group that received the vitamin—with no evidence of toxicity.

Carotene should also be included in any supplement program to boost immunity. Not only is carotene a potent antioxidant, but it also appears to help protect us against many forms of cancer.

Vitamin C Is Crucial to Immunity

Vitamin C is so vital to immunity that no campaign to strengthen your defenses against infectious diseases should be without it. Vitamin C boosts the activity of the lymphocytes and macrophages (large cells that devour invaders), and raises levels of interferon (an infection-fighting biochemical). Vitamin C also has specific effects in strengthening our response to viral infections. These effects have been duplicated by different researchers time and time again in human experiments. In my clinical practice (MR), I have seen vitamin C work wonders of boosting immune power. I must confess, however, that some people seem to respond better to vitamin A than to vitamin C. The point is that the media have promoted vitamin C as an immunity-boosting nutrient, which it certainly is. However, many people neglect vitamin A and other immune boosters. When they start on a comprehensive immune-strengthening program such as this one, they get much better results than when they were simply taking high doses of vitamin C.

The bioflavonoids are also important boosters of the immune system. They have demonstrated the ability to increase the body's defenses against viruses, bacteria, and fungi. Apparently, bioflavonoids strengthen the immune system in more than one way. By reducing inflammation and allergic responses, they leave the immune system stronger to fight infections. They are also known to deactivate enzymes that produce symptoms in viral infections.

Bioflavonoids also boost the effectiveness of vitamin C. Not only do they increase the body's utilization of vitamin C, but they also preserve the vitamin from oxidation and conversion, thus making it more available to the tissues. In combination with vitamin C, bioflavonoids can reduce the healing time of herpes sores on the lips by as much as two-thirds.

Vitamin E and Selenium Directly Boost Immunity

Vitamin E serves the immune system in many ways. First of all, it is a potent antioxidant, so it helps protect the immune system against damage from its own weapons, the free radicals.

Most people know about vitamin E's antioxidant powers. But few people—including physicians—know that vitamin E is also a direct stimulant of the immune system. Increasing vitamin E intake above normal dietary amounts results in direct stimulation and strengthening of the body's ability to produce antibodies, thus significantly increasing resistance. The invader-devouring phagocytes are also directly stimulated. The boosting is magnified further if small amounts of selenium are included along with the vitamin E. Selenium is important not only as an antioxidant, but also as a stimulant to the immune system, together with vitamin E.

Zinc—The Primary Immune Factor

Zinc, a mineral that exists only in borderline amounts in the American diet, is crucial to the effectiveness of the immune system. A zinc deficiency is known to speed up the atrophy of the thymus gland and reduce thymosin levels and the number of T cells. Like vitamins A, E, C, and selenium, zinc is a potent immunostimulant. Zinc also speeds healing after surgery or injury.

Vitamin B_6 (pyridoxine) and zinc boost each other's effects on the immune system. Another B vitamin, folic acid, is also required to maintain immune strength. Pantothenic acid has always been known as the B vitamin most important to our response to stress. But how many people know that when this vitamin is deficient, the immune response —particularly the response to viral and bacterial infection —is compromised? Circulating antibodies drop significantly when pantothenic acid or pyridoxine are deficient.

Immune Booster from Japan

The mineral germanium, a brand new supplement in the United States, is a potent immune booster. Germanium stimulates the body's production of interferon, which fights viral infections and abnormal cell growths. We believe that germanium has additional immune-strengthening powers as well. If you have difficulty finding germanium supplements, you can still get germanium by taking garlic. Garlic contains very high concentrations of this mineral, perhaps explaining garlic's effectiveness as an immune stimulant.

Enzymes Are Immune Accelerators

Enzymes that are known to digest protein molecules are also effective boosters of the immune system. Trypsin (produced by the pancreas), papain (raw papaya), and bromelain (raw pineapple) are three principal proteases (protein-digesting enzymes). These enzymes speed up the production of lymphocytes in the bone marrow.

Amino Acids Maintain Immune Strength

Growth hormone (GH) is the body's own way of retaining youth, because it helps maintain the thymus gland. This pituitary hormone is normally released when we sleep, exercise, fast, have low blood sugar, and are under the influence of certain drugs (dopaminergic stimulants). Some research shows that after age thirty normal exercise no longer stimulates GH release, and that only sustained peak exercise—not long, slow exercise—is beneficial. Nevertheless, intake of the amino acids arginine and ornithine also stimulates GH release.

Arginine not only stimulates GH, but also boosts the T cells and the body's general metabolism. Arginine, by supporting a strong thymus gland, prevents weakening of the immune system caused by stress. Ornithine also strengthens the T cells.

Lysine boost the body's production of antiviral agents and speeds healing of herpes viral sores. High levels of lysine in the cell inhibit viral growth and reproduction. Lysine has been used effectively in preventing the outbreak of genital herpes sores. In order to be effective, however, the diet must not be high in arginine. This means that if you want to take lysine for the prevention of herpes outbreaks, you must not take arginine and you must reduce the level of arginine in your diet by decreasing your intake of nuts, seeds, chocolate, and grains.

Taurine performs a critical role within the white blood cells. It boosts the phagoctyes' ability to destroy bacteria. Taurine may be especially effective in strengthening the body's resistance against *Candida* infections.

Glutathione also enhances the activity of the white blood cells, particularly the phagocytes, whose job it is to devour invading molecules and microorganisms. Glutathione also combines with selenium to form glutathione peroxidase, one of the body's own free radical scavengers. Glutathione also helps increase the effectiveness of vitamin C, by converting the oxidized vitamin back to its effective form.

The "outlaw vitamin" also comes through for the immune system. DMG (dimethylglycine) is also a potent immune stimulant. It can boost the antibody response by a factor of four and the white blood cell response by a factor of three.

The Right Amounts
of the Right Oils Are Essential

Essential fatty acids are also required for a healthy immune system. As we described earlier, gamma-linolenic acid is converted to PG1 series prostaglandins, which support immune strength. (As an example of how nutrients interact and support one another: vitamin C, niacin, folic acid, pyridoxine, zinc, and magnesium are all required for the conversion of gamma-linolenic acid to the PG1 prostaglandins.) When PG1 prostaglandins are high, immune power is boosted. Because the PG1 prostaglandins are anti-inflammatory, however, raising them too high could depress the immune system. As in the case of zinc, which can also depress the immune system when taken in excess, this is a case of too much of a good thing working the opposite effect. In our immune supplement, we include a basic essential fatty supplement in the form of evening primrose oil. Any other oil supplying gamma-linolenic acid, such as black currant seed oil, could also be substituted.

Glandulars Keep the Immune System Young

Among the glandular supplements, thymus substance is the most important. You want all the possible rejuvenation of the thymus gland that you can get, because the thymus gland is the major controlling gland of the immune system. It is a "teacher" gland that instructs immune warriors how to select and destroy enemy organisms and foreign invaders. The thymus gland, unfortunately, shrinks as we grow older. Properly prepared thymus concentrate contains thymosin, the hormone that "teaches" the immune system. Thymus extract has been used successfully to boost immune power in persons with weakened immunity. Thymosin does not have to survive digestion in order to be effective; fragments of the hormone entering the bloodstream are sufficient to stimulate immune strength.

Thymus substance may also provide substances that can regenerate thymosin within the body. Zinc is also important to the body's supply of thymosin. Thymulin, a form of thymosin also known as thymus factor, is a small protein that is absorbable through the intestinal wall. Thymus factor requires adequate zinc levels in order to function.

Spleen extract may also be used as an immune stimulant. The spleen is the largest lymphoid organ in the body, and it cooperates with the thymus as a part of the immune system. White blood cells and other cells that consume and destroy invaders are formed and stored in the spleen. When needed, these white blood cells are discharged en masse. We know that vigorous exercise can double the number of white blood cells in the blood.

Injected spleen extract has been used since 1929 for support and stimulation of the immune system, specifically in the treatment of people with Hodgkin's disease. It can boost lymphatic activity throughout the entire body. Injected spleen extract has an antiviral action similar to interferon and is also capable of detoxifying bacterial toxins. Spleen extract or concentrate may also contain thymus-stimulating factors, and may not only heal spleen and bone marrow, but also enhance resistance to abnormal cell growth. Spleen concentrate has anti-inflammatory and antiblood-clotting properties as well.

Spleen substance may also help protect us from radiation. In animal experiments, spleen extract speeds the recovery of the spleen, bone marrow, skin, and thymus gland after radiation exposure.

Next, thyroid substance should be included for its power to stimulate the entire immune system. Thyroid substance can nudge a sluggish thyroid gland and stimulate the bone marrow to produce ample quantities of lymphocytes.

Finally, adrenal substance should be included in your immune supplement. The adrenal glands are central to the body's response to any kind of stress, including infections. When the adrenals are at an ebb, the immune system is not primed for an adequate defense.

Beyond Vitamins Multisupplement
to Boost Immunity

For additional information on how to design your personal
Beyond Vitamins Program, see Chapter 15.

VITAMINS
Vitamin A	25,000 I.U.
Carotene	25,000 I.U.
Pyridoxine	50 mg.
Pantothenic acid	100–1,000 mg.
Folic acid	800–2,000 mcg.
Vitamin C	2,000–10,000 mg.
Bioflavonoids	1,000–2,000 mg.
Vitamin E	400–800 I.U.

MINERALS
Selenium	100–200 mcg.
Zinc	30–100 mg.

AMINO ACIDS
Lysine	1,000 mg. (before breakfast)
Glutathione	200 mg.
Ornithine	1,000–2,000 mg.
Arginine	1,000–3,000 mg.
Taurine	100–500 mg.
Trypsin	100 mg.
Papain	100 mg.
Bromelain	100 mg.

GLANDULARS
Adrenal	50 mg.
Spleen	50 mg.
Thymus	50 mg.
Thyroid	50 mg.

OTHERS
DMG	100–200 mg.
GLA (EPO)	40 mg (500 mg. EPO)
Germanium	100 mg.

CHAPTER
6 Feel Younger Longer

IF YOU STUDY the healthy human body up to about age twenty, you will come away convinced that it is designed to last at least two or three times longer than it actually does. No machine made by humans is able to heal itself, defend itself against microscopic invaders, and regenerate itself despite constant wear and tear.

Yet something happens when we're in our twenties. The wear and tear, the stress and strain, begin to catch up with us. When we're young, the balance between wear and tear and growth and repair is in our favor. The body holds its own and is able to regenerate new tissue, create energy, and defend itself against disease. But then the balance slowly starts to shift.

Even then, the balance is strongly in our favor for many more years. Besides aging itself, only severe illness, injury, or trauma of some kind can upset that balance. But once that balance is upset far enough, almost all of our body functions begin to deteriorate. Nothing works as well as it did when we were younger.

Many of the nutrients we've been discussing in this book can help us keep the balance in our favor. Other chapters in the Beyond Vitamins Program have been concerned with preventing or healing illness and injury, and with boosting performance. This chapter deals with aging itself.

Of course, we can't talk about aging without talking abut disease also. Degenerative disease, particularly cardiovascular disease, diabetes, and arthritis, are not only symptoms of aging—they're also causes of aging.

In addition to degenerative diseases, the other causes of aging are:

- Stress
- Accumulation of toxins
- Free radicals
- Cross-linking of molecules
- Errors in our DNA
- Autoimmunity
- Changes in the brain
- The aging clock

None of these causes of aging are independent of the others; they all overlap to a great degree. Although we know that they all play a role, we don't understand exactly why they occur. Of all of them, the greatest mystery surrounds the working of the aging clock, whose very existence is highly controversial.

We'll explain a little about each one and then tell you about some nutrients that can help offset these factors and keep the balance in our favor. Because we've already talked about stress, toxins, and free radicals, we'll begin with the role disease plays in aging.

DEGENERATIVE DISEASES MAKE US OLDER

A very high proportion of the symptoms we usually associate with aging are caused by degenerative diseases. When we lose the ability to run up stairs, hills, or streets the way we did when we were kids, we don't say we feel ill, we say we feel older.

When our joints ache for no good reason other than the fact that we got out of bed, we feel older.

When we can't see or hear or make love as much or as intensely as we did when we were young, we feel older.

We tend to think of the major degenerative disease, cardiovascular disease, as a life-and-death disease. There's no question that it is a matter of life and death. But long before it kills, cardiovascular disease impairs the circulation a little at a time. And as it does, it ages us.

Our organs and glands depend on the circulation of blood to carry life-giving oxygen and nutrients and carry away toxic by-products. When the flow of blood is impaired, so is the ability of the organ or gland to do its job.

Most people think of their blood vessels as a kind of human plumbing. Actually, the veins, arteries, and capillaries are better than metal or plastic pipes, because they help move the blood along by pulsing with the flow. As we get older, however, the blood vessels gradually lose their elasticity and their ability to pulse. As a result, the blood moves more turbulently against the walls, increasing the wear and tear on them. Blood pressure increases, and the heart has to work harder. At stress points along the system, little smooth muscle tumors develop and fatty deposits accumulate around them.

We don't know all the reasons why these fatty deposits accumulate. But we do know that the clotting tendencies of the blood, the amount of easily oxidized, rancid oils, and the amount of sugar in the diet are all factors. The tiny smooth muscle tumors around which the fatty deposits accumulate occur at places where the cell wall has been damaged by free radical oxidation and turbulent blood flow. An excess of cholesterol and unstable oils in the diet makes these tumors and fatty deposits more likely to occur. A high sugar diet also causes the fatty deposits by stimulating excess secretion of insulin, which also tends to give rise to fatty deposits.

NUTRIENTS THAT HELP PREVENT DEGENERATIVE DISEASE

Vitamin A and beta-carotene are first-line nutritional defenses against degenerative disease, especially cancer. Repeated scientific studies have shown that high levels of vitamin A and carotene in the diet significantly lessen the risk of many forms of cancer.

Vitamin C strengthens the blood vessels and helps remove cholesterol from the body, thus helping to lower our risk of cardiovascular disease. Vitamin C may help prevent cancer by strengthening the immune system, particularly those parts of the immune system that destroy abnormal cell growths.

Vitamin E has long been known to help prevent cardiovascular disease by reducing the tendency of the blood to form dangerous clots, which can block the flow of blood to vital organs.

BIOFLAVONOIDS DEACTIVATE AGING

Bioflavonoids may one day be the treatment of choice for cataracts, because they can deactivate the enzyme, aldose reductase, which causes some types of cataracts—particularly those most common in diabetics. The enzyme converts blood sugar (which is often abnormally high in diabetics) into sorbitol, which accumulates and crystallizes in the lens of the eye. Not only do the sorbitol crystals affect the transmission of light through the lens, but they also soak up water and cause increased pressure and tissue damage. In animal experiments, bioflavonoid supplements inhibit the development of diabetic cataracts.

Bioflavonoids not only deactivate potentially harmful enzymes, but they also stimulate helpful ones. They are known to boost the activity of certain enzymes that inactivate and convert toxic, cancer-causing pollutants into forms that can be safely excreted from the body.

A NEW ANTI-CANCER ROLE
FOR CALCIUM

Calcium has only recently been identified as a nutrient that can help prevent cancer, especially colorectal cancer. In this form of cancer, the normal balance between abnormal cell growth and normal growth in the bowel shifts to favor abnormal growth. Calcium can actually reduce abnormal cell growth in the bowel and restore equilibrium to the extent that the bowels of high-risk people more closely resemble those of low-risk people.

Calcium is also a factor in preventing cardiovascular disease by lowering blood pressure. Several recent studies have pointed out that low levels of calcium in the diet can lead to high blood pressure, and high calcium levels seem to offer some protection. In one study, calcium supplements were effective in lowering blood pressure in women with high blood pressure, whereas it had no effect in women with normal blood pressure.

A BRIGHT STAR AMONG MINERALS

When it comes to helping prevent degenerative disease, chromium is the mineral that really shines. One of the reasons that we have so much cardiovascular disease is the high level of sugar in our diet. Sugar and other sweets upset our body's glucose (blood sugar) tolerance mechanisms. Too much insulin is secreted to deal with all the sugar, and the excess insulin is believed to damage the blood vessels. Chromium helps in this area because it is a cofactor for insulin, and increases the efficiency of the hormone, thus making less of it necessary to control blood sugar. When chromium levels in the blood rise, circulating insulin levels fall, and vice versa. Because chromium is so effective, it improves glucose tolerance in diabetics as well as nondiabetics.

But that's not all chromium does. Chromium is also partly responsible for the metabolism of fats, so a chromium deficiency weakens the body's ability to metabolize fats effectively, including cholesterol. A chromium deficiency can raise blood levels of cholesterol. Raising dietary levels of chromium can lower blood levels of cholesterol, and raise HDL levels, which indicate that cholesterol is being properly metabolized and discarded by the body.

Low chromium levels in diet and blood are now considered major risk factors for cardiovascular disease and diabetes. This fact is all the more important when you realize that the USDA admits that most Americans are not getting adequate chromium in their diets. Not only is chromium removed by most food processing, but it is used up and excreted by the body in higher concentrations when we exercise, undergo stress, and eat sweets. Runners, for example, excrete twice as much chromium on days when they run as on days they don't run.

Raising dietary levels of chromium is more than insurance against degenerative disease. Chromium improves glucose tolerance, which translates into more energy and stamina.

Selenium is another major antidegenerative disease nutrient. Over the years there have been repeated studies showing that adequate selenium levels in the diet lower our risk of cancer and cardiovascular disease.

Magnesium plays more than one role in preventing cardiovascular disease. As a mineral that, together with calcium, controls muscle tension and nerve irritability, magnesium can lower blood pressure. Magnesium is also vital to maintaining normal heart rhythm.

DEFUSE STRESS WITH TRYPTOPHAN

The amino acid tryptophan may also be useful in preventing cardiovascular disease. Tryptophan not only lowers blood pressure in people with high blood pressure, but it also lowers LDL cholesterol and raises HDL cholesterol. Using tryptophan for these purposes may be especially useful for tense, nervous, anxious people who tend to have depression or insomnia. Tryptophan can be used as a tranquilizer, which will not only help induce sleep when taken at night, but relieve depression when taking during the day.

As with any tranquilizer, even a natural one such as tryptophan, we urge you not to become dependent on regular use, but rather to use the tranquilizer to give you a respite from your symptoms, a respite that will allow you to explore the reasons why you are nervous, tense, anxious, or depressed.

EPA-containing fish oils offer us help with two degenerative diseases—arthritis and cardiovascular disease. The studies that began to draw all the attention to fish oils established EPA as a major factor in preventing cardiovascular disease. People with high levels of EPA have less risk of developing cardiovascular disease. EPA in fish oils stimulates the production of anti-inflammatory prostaglandins, which lower blood pressure, widen the blood vessels, reduce the tendency of the blood to clot, and decrease the inflammation in the blood vessels, which leads to atherosclerosis.

EPA, or fish oil, also helps relieve arthritis. A daily supplement of fish oil providing EPA can relieve tender joints, morning stiffness, and fatigue in rheumatoid arthritis. EPA works best when it is combined with a low-fat diet. That means a diet low in all fat, not just animal fats. Polyunsaturated fats, vegetable oils, and margarine must also be reduced. When these oils and fats are used to excess—and most of us do use them to excess—they can stimulate the production of inflammatory prostaglandins, which over-whelm the anti-inflammatory prostaglandins produced by EPA.

MUCOPOLYSACCHARIDES, THE CUTTING EDGE OF CVD PREVENTION

Mucopolysaccharides may be difficult to pronounce and even a bigger challenge to spell, but in years to come they may well be making headlines as major anti-aging supplements. Some very exciting research has investigated the role played by mucopolysaccharides in preventing cardio-vascular disease. The wall of the artery contains high amounts of mucopolysaccharides, which appear to help strengthen the artery. Whether or not blood fats ever begin to take hold in the wall of the artery seems to depend on the amount and quality of mucopolysaccharides present.

Do supplements of mucopolysaccharides actually protect against cardiovascular disease? We do know that supplements do lengthen the clotting time of the blood—a very important risk factor in cardiovascular disease. Moreover, because mucopolysaccharides do appear to reduce inflammation by strengthening the membranes, we believe supplements (which are also available as chondroitan sulfate A, or CSA) may prove to be an important part of a total program to resist aging, stress, and degenerative disease.

CROSS-LINKING OF MOLECULES— THE DEADLY SQUARE DANCE

These mischievous bonds between normally free mole-cules not only damage large molecules, such as the proteins and nucleic acids of the connective tissue, but they also damage small molecules, such as the DNA and RNA. Once joined in this way, the molecules are severely hampered in their ability to carry out their specific functions. Cross-links attack the very foundation of the connective tissue of the body, collagen, and slowly reduce the flexibility of skin and blood vessels—the whole body. Avenues of circulation are choked off. Nutrients can't get through to strangled tissue, waste products that cannot be removed accumulate and worsen the toxic effect.

Cross-linking contributes to cardiovascular disease, cancer, diabetes, weakened muscles, autoimmune disorders such as arthritis, wrinkled skin, high blood pressure, and many other health problems.

When cross-linking occurs in the genes, incorrect genetic information is passed on and further damage is done. (We will explain this further in the next section.)

Cross-links can be caused by free radicals, which form the unwelcome bridges between normally unattached molecules. Thus anything that generates free radicals will also increase cross-linking, including air pollution and other environmental toxins, radiation, smoke, metabolites of alcohol, heavy metal pollutants such as cadmium, lead, and aluminum, and sunlight. Toxic by-products the body itself creates during periods of stress, illness, and exhaustion are also potent agents of cross-linking.

NUTRIENTS THAT
RESIST CROSS-LINKING

Because cross-links are caused by free radicals, all of the nutrients that reduce free radicals will also help slow down the formation of cross-links. (For a discussion of these nutrients, the antioxidants, see Chapter 4. When designing your personal supplement program at the end of this book, include the column for Stress Supplements to ensure that you do not miss any specific nutrients. Doing this will also ensure the correct dose ranges for overlapping supplements.)

In addition, protein-digesting enzymes such as bromelain and papaya are capable of digesting and eliminating cross-links. Although they are not very potent, they may help somewhat.

Protecting the skin against ultraviolet radiation from sunlight is the best way to protect the skin from becoming leathery and wrinkled from cross-linking. Beta-carotene, the vitamin A precursor, can also help protect the skin from sunlight.

WHEN OUR DNA FORGETS, WE GET OLDER

DNA does not control growth only when we're developing in the womb. Throughout life, DNA provides the blueprint for all growth and repair. RNA molecules serve as the "foremen" who deliver the DNA messages to the protein-manufacturing assembly line of the cells. As we age, however, this blueprint becomes distorted and the messengers begin to misrepresent their messages. Some of this distortion is caused by free radicals and cross-links, which scribble in new lines in the blueprint and erase old ones.

A certain percentage of the distortions may simply be random errors among the billions of DNA-RNA interchanges. We know that RNA levels tend to decrease with age, and that the remaining RNA is more likely to make errors in transmitting messages to the cells. Finally, there is a theory that the tendency to distort the DNA-RNA messages controlling growth and repair is actually built in to the gene itself. (This theory overlaps with the "aging clock" theory, which we'll discuss later.)

Distorted genetic messages cause a lot of trouble. Because of these faulty instructions, the cells will manufacture faulty proteins, enzymes, and hormones that are less effective—and even harmful. The immune system may be primed to attack these faulty proteins, wasting its vital resources and harming functional tissues at the same time.

As more and more faulty proteins are created, they become a drain on the body's resources.

NUTRIENTS THAT
HELP OUR DNA REMEMBER

All of the antioxidants will help maintain the DNA and RNA by helping to neutralize free radicals and prevent cross-linking (see Chapter 4).

Essential amino acids supplied by high-quality protein foods or amino acid supplements should also help to offset the deterioration of the DNA. When the body is deficient in essential amino acids, protein synthesis is faulty, with or without errors in DNA.

Vitamin C, choline, riboflavin, folic acid, biotin, pantothenic acid, B_6, zinc, manganese, and chromium are all required for the maintenance of correct DNA and RNA.

What is perhaps the most important method of preserving accurate DNA and RNA is the use of nucleic acids, which are required for the construction of DNA and RNA. A diet high in nucleic acids supplies the body's DNA and RNA with fresh raw material for constructing new DNA and RNA. Nucleic acids are highest in brewer's yeast and sardines. Plant foods supply only RNA, whereas animal foods supply both RNA and DNA.

We also believe that glandular supplements are high in nucleic acids and that may be one reason to include these supplements in a total youth extension supplement program. Later in this chapter, we have included a special section on glandulars.

AUTOIMMUNITY—WHEN OUR BODYGUARD TURNS AGAINST US

Autoimmune aging is easy to understand: The army that has been defending the body so well for the first 20 to 30 years of life slowly begins to turn around and attack its own home. The immune system's "vision" clouds and it loses the ability to distinguish "self" from "not self." As a result, "self" is sometimes attacked and "not self" isn't.

The autoimmune consequences may include rheumatoid arthritis, systemic lupus, multiple sclerosis, some forms of anemia and kidney disease, and increased susceptibility to all infections and diseases normally resisted by the immune system.

This gradual decline in the efficiency of the immune system is caused by many factors: the ubiquitous free radicals, cross-links, "slow" viral infections that confuse the immune system, inherited or aging-related distortions of the DNA, the slow ticking of the "aging clock" and, perhaps most important, the degeneration of the thymus gland, the gland that is responsible for "teaching" important segments of our immune army how—and what—to fight.

NUTRIENTS TO HELP KEEP OUR IMMUNE SYSTEM ON OUR SIDE

To resist immune aging, the nutrients we described in Chapter 5 on boosting immunity will help maintain the strength of the system. When designing your personal program in Chapter 15, please include the column of Immunity supplements. This will ensure that your dose ranges will be correct and you will not miss any valuable supplements.

CHANGES IN THE BRAIN
AGE US ALL OVER

"It's all in your head" doesn't mean quite the same thing it once did. Years ago, when somebody told you a problem you had was "all in your head," it was a way of dismissing the problem as merely caused by the imagination. Today we know better. We know that thinking, imagination, and other brain functions are, if not controlled, then at least encouraged or discouraged by the biochemical environment of the brain. Moreover, we know that thoughts "in your head" can also influence many aspects of your physical condition.

Everything the brain does is modulated by neurotransmitters that regulate the passage of impulses over gaps between the nerve cells. The balance of these neurotransmitters has a great deal of power over the function of the brain. If certain neurotransmitters are on the upswing, so will our mood be up. If others are predominant, we may become depressed.

NUTRIENTS THAT KEEP
OUR BRAIN ON-LINE

The bad news is that as we get older, the balance of neurotransmitters starts to change. The good news is that the balance of many of the most important neurotransmitters can be affected by our diet.

For example, acetylcholine is the neurotransmitter that regulates the entire parasympathetic nervous system, which includes the actions of the muscles, memory, learning, secretions, and excretion of waste products from the bowel and bladder. Acetylcholine is also used by the primitive parts of the brain that control emotions, reflexes, instincts, sex drive, and alertness. When our acetylcholine levels in the brain dip, we start forgetting things, grow irritable more easily, have trouble concentrating and sleeping, become uncoordinated, and lose interest in sex. Choline is a dietary precursor of acetylcholine. High dietary amounts of choline can raise brain levels of acetylcholine. Choline supplements (phosphatidyl choline, from lecithin) have been used to improve memory and other mental functions in the aged. Choline can also help boost mental function, especially memory, in younger people

Norepinephrine is the neurotransmitter that regulates walking and running, aggression, sex drive, appetite, and other mental functions. Dopamine is another stimulatory neurotransmitter, closely related to norepinephrine. As we get older, levels of these neurotransmitters, known as the catecholamines, begin to decline. Depression, apathy, and loss of sex drive may result. The amino acids phenylalanine and tyrosine are used by the brain to make catecholamines.

Serotonin is an inhibitory neurotransmitter. Whereas the catecholamines and acetylcholine stimulate the transmission of nerve impulses, serotonin stimulates nerve cells that reduce brain activity. When serotonin levels start to fall, we may become agitated or have trouble falling asleep. The amino acid tryptophan raises brain levels of serotonin and is very effective in helping to induce sleep. It has also been used successfully to treat certain agitated forms of depression.

THE MYSTERIOUS AGING CLOCK

The aging clock is used to explain all the causes of aging that we don't yet understand. After all the random and accidental causes of aging are examined, there still seems to be a limiting factor somehow built into the body, which ages us. Some theories hold that the aging clock is within the cell, and that the cells of the body can reproduce only a limited number of times. Some theories state that the aging clock exists in the DNA molecule, which purposely transmits faulty information once we have lived enough time to bear offspring (and pass on our genes). Other theories state that the aging clock is in the brain or the endocrine system, and that a "death hormone" is secreted, which stimulates all of the age-related deterioration in structure and function.

Someday we may be able to find and reset our aging clock. Right now, we don't know enough about the aging clock to even find it, let alone reset it. All we can do is try to deal with the effects, by using the nutrients described in earlier sections of this chapter. Aside from these supplementary methods, the only other method that shows some promise is the use of high-nutrient-density, low-calorie diet. In animal experiments, cutting calories by 20 percent so that weight stabilizes at around 80 percent of normal can double life span. In certain isolated human societies where the average daily intake is from 1,200 to 1,900 calories, people do appear to live longer.

We do not recommend drastically cutting caloric intake unless the diet is carefully designed to provide a high density of nutrients and adequate protein. The Beyond Vitamins Multisupplement for weight loss (Chapter 8) contains information about supplements for people on a low-calorie diet.

As part of our Beyond Vitamins supplement program, we have included glandular supplements. Because glandular supplements derive most of their scientific justification from the same sources as cell therapy, a very popular method of youth extension, we have saved our discussion of glandular therapy for this chapter.

CELL THERAPY IN A BOTTLE—
FOR 1/500 THE COST

Glandular extracts have had a long and somewhat checkered history. They were among the original cornerstones of medicine, and were first used many thousands of years ago. Most ancient cultures, from the Egyptians, to the Hindus, to the Greeks, used glandular therapy. They worked under the assumption that "like heals like," or that an ailing human organ or gland could be healed by administering tissue from the same organ or gland (from an animal). Down through the ages this has meant either injecting the tissue, implanting it surgically, or taking it orally.

In the nineteenth century, medical science discovered glandular secretions that could, in very small amounts, exert powerful effects on the body. These secretions, named hormones, were extracted from their respective glands and used as drugs to regenerate and heal. This form of glandular therapy prospers today under the conventional sanctions of hormonal replacement therapy, except that, today, the hormones are synthesized rather than extracted from glands.

HORMONES ARE NOT THE GLANDS'
ONLY ACTIVE INGREDIENTS

Around the turn of the century, while most physicians were using glandular therapy in the form of hormonal extracts, others were not satisfied that the hormones were the only substances in glands to have a stimulating effect. Although legitimate research was carried out in hopes of discovering these healing substances, some practices may have wandered over the border between experimentation and opportunism.

For example, some enterprising "surgeons" (at least one was actually a barber), performed thousands of "goat gland" and "monkey gland" operations supposedly to restore or boost male sexual potency. Tissue from the testes of goats and other animals was surgically implanted, or grafted, in hopes of lending the operation's human recipients the legendary sexual potency of the goat.

It didn't take long for the operation to fall into disrepute. Nevertheless, respectable scientists continued research into various forms of glandular therapy.

THE BIRTH OF CELL THERAPY

In 1931, Swiss physician Paul Niehans developed a form of glandular therapy that is still practiced and officially recognized in Europe. Niehans was called to try to save the life of a woman whose parathyroid gland was removed by accident during an operation. Recognizing the extreme urgency of the situation—and knowing that there was nothing conventional medicine could do for the woman—he injected a whole diced parathyroid gland from a freshly slaughtered sheep into the woman's bloodstream. Even to Niehans's surprise, the woman not only survived, but went on to live a vigorous life until in her nineties. Niehans's assumption was that the injection stimulated the regeneration of the woman's parathyroid gland.

Niehans went on to develop what he called "cell therapy," or "live cell therapy," at his clinic in Switzerland. The rich, famous, and powerful from all over the world flocked to his clinic to receive injections of fetal glandular tissue (from sheep), in hopes of rejuvenating their own aging organs and glands. The rationale for the treatment was that somehow, the cells from the injected glandular tissue found their way to the specific tissue in the human body and, once there, were able to stimulate a healing or rejuvenation of the diseased or worn out organ or gland.

Niehans used cell therapy not only for youth extension, but also in the specific treatment of illness. He cultivated the concept of "like heals like" into a comprehensive medical practice.

CELL THERAPY IS ACCEPTED IN EUROPE

Cell therapy was eventually accepted by physicians all over Europe. Presently, cell therapy is not only legal in Europe, but is paid for by the government health plans of several countries. You can obtain cell therapy in most countries in Europe. Or, if you have $5,000 or more to spend, you can go to the glamorous clinic Niehans himself built.

Or, for about 1/500 the cost, you can treat yourself using raw glandular supplements, which, many people believe, work on the same principal as Niehans's cell therapy. Oral glandular therapy is definitely safer. The threat of a severe allergic reaction shocking the system is practically eliminated when the glandular extract is taken orally rather than injected.

Today, glandular therapy is highly controversial. On the one hand it is controversial in the same way that other nutritional therapies are, because it is different from modern medicine's way of doing things. While Niehans was developing cell therapy, pharmaceutical research was learning how to synthesize hormones. Thus hormonal replacement therapy became part of high-tech, modern medicine. The split with glandular therapy was then almost complete.

But even among nutritionally oriented physicians, glandular supplements are controversial. Though "like heals like" is a very appealing concept, it is almost too simplistic, too "magical" for our contemporary, scientifically trained attitudes. In our opinion, however, it's not the simplicity of the concept that makes glandulars controversial, it's the fact that, despite its apparent simplicity, we just don't know enough to understand how it might work. Ignorance is usually the first cause of denial and disagreement.

THE SCIENCE BEHIND GLANDULAR THERAPY

Actually, as magical as "like heals like" may appear, the concept is valid. It does work, and modern medicine does use it. If you asked a conventional physician what he or she thinks of glandular therapy, or of the concept behind it, you'd most likely see the physician's head shake in disbelief and hear it dismissed as one of the fads of the lunatic fringe.

But if you asked the physician what he or she thought of bone marrow transplants, such as the kind performed by American physicians on the victims of the Chernobyl nuclear accident, the physician would nod and agree that the wonders of modern medicine were truly amazing.

A bone marrow transplant, such as the ones celebrated in the press as an example of Western medicine's superiority, consists of first obtaining bone marrow from within the hip of a human donor with blood and tissue types that closely match the recipient. The bone marrow is then injected into the bloodstream of the recipient, where it finds its way to the recipient's own bone marrow. The purpose of the transplant is to rejuvenate bone marrow that has been damaged (in this case by radiation). The new bone marrow is able to stimulate the damaged bone marrow to repair itself and resume its vital role as manufacturer of blood cells. To us, that sounds remarkably like the very process Niehans described: Like heals like.

The average conventional physician would probably scoff at the notion that brain or adrenal concentrates could have any beneficial effects on human brain function. But, on the forefront of modern medical research, surgeons are grafting brain and adrenal tissue onto the diseased brains of sufferers of Parkinson's disease, and observing some improvement in symptoms. Shades of those "goat gland" and "monkey gland" operations!

So the concept behind glandular therapy is definitely neither nonscientific nor foolhardy. It forms the basis of some of modern medicine's most highly regarded procedures and innovative research.

Nevertheless, when applied to nutritional supplementation with glandular tissues, the concept is controversial. But we are finding out more and more about how glandular therapy might work, and there is evidence that it does, indeed, work in several instances.

POTENT CELL STIMULATORS DO SURVIVE

One of the principal controversies regarding glandular supplements concerns whether any active glandular substance is able to survive the human digestive process and be absorbed into the bloodstream in a form that might be effective. There is evidence that extremely minute amounts of certain very potent substances do make their way into the bloodstream, and that these substances can stimulate specific organs or glands to restore lost function or rebuild worn or destroyed tissue.

We know that pancreatic extract supplements can be remarkably effective in improving digestion and absorption. Tests have shown that small amounts of the pancreatic enzymes survive the acid medium of the stomach and pass into the intestine, where they boost digestion in persons with severe pancreatic insufficiency.

There is a mystery, however: The supplements supply only about 5 to 10 percent of the amount of pancreatic enzymes the body normally uses, although this amount is as effective as a full dose. Scientists do not understand how such a relatively small amount of surviving enzymes can exert such a powerful effect on digestion.

We also know that some of these pancreatic enzymes enter the bloodstream, where they can exert a local or systemic anti-inflammatory effect. It is possible that, along with these enzymes, some of these small, but potent, hormonelike substances are also carried into the bloodstream, where they travel to the pancreas and stimulate normal secretion? We don't know.

But we do know that glands do "communicate" and stimulate each other by means other than hormones. The pituitary gland, for example, secretes small "messenger" proteins that stimulate specific target glands and organs. These messenger substances are so potent that the effective dose may weigh less than 1/1000 the weight of the period at the end of this sentence.

POWERFUL MESSENGERS AT WORK

One such messenger substance is currently in use as a prescription drug. Extracted from the hypothalamus of the brain, Hypothalamus Releasing Factor (HRF) is used to treat certain types of depression, insomnia, anxiety, and behavior problems. HRF stimulates the pituitary to release its own messenger substances, which then balance endocrine levels and restore balance in the glands and in the brain. Two facts are important: First, HRF treatments need not be prolonged. A short course of therapy restores balance for many months afterward, much like Niehans claimed cell therapy worked. Second, although HRF is usually given by injection, it is capable of surviving the gastrointestinal tract and being absorbed into the bloodstream.

In another classic experiment, Ershoff demonstrated that liver extract was able to improve performance and resistance to stress and disease—over and above what was stimulated by the known vitamins and minerals supplied by liver. Were these messenger substances at work? Again, we don't know for sure.

Ershoff wasn't the first to find therapeutic effects for liver. A 1929 study demonstrated that when diabetics ate ½ pound of liver three or four times each week, they reduced or eliminated their insulin requirement. This effect was most likely caused by the liver's high levels of glucose-tolerance-factor chromium. However, rejuvenation of the liver's ability to support energy metabolism is also possible.

Other studies have found that heart substance (or even cooked heart muscle) can improve sugar metabolism and general muscular activity.

Glandular supplements are foods, not drugs. The elements present in glandulars may be just as necessary as vitamins, minerals, amino acids, essential oils, and other nutrients, and just as much a part of the natural food diet our bodies are designed to thrive on. If glandulars—and other Beyond Vitamin supplements—boost our general health, strength, stamina, vigor, and mental performance, they may simply be restoring the body to its natural condition. Glandulars are a difficult area because we truly do not know enough to isolate and identify all the specific substances that may be at work. For some people that may be enough to condemn or ignore glandular therapy. For others it's a cloak under which they feel free to make wild, perhaps fraudulent, claims. Some people say glandulars are useless; some say they are panaceas.

We have presented this information about glandulars to enable you to make up your own mind, to let you know that the truth lies somewhere in between, and that there is a reasonable, hopeful place between the two extremes. We also provide this information, as we do all the information in this book, hoping that you will find it useful and that it will stimulate you to further explore the ways in which food substances can help us lead longer, better lives. Because the tiny "messenger" proteins in glandulars are so powerful, we advise care and caution in the use of glandular supplements.

So in our Beyond Vitamins Multisupplement for Youth

Extension, we are including a complete glandular supplement as an option.

MAKE SURE YOU ABSORB YOUR FOOD!

The last anti-aging supplement we're going to describe may be the most important: digestive enzymes. As we get older, our hydrochloric acid and digestive enzymes begin to decline. You might consider this a result of the aging clock's mischief. The reduction in digestive efficiency results in a gradual decrease in absorption of vital nutrients. This begins an ever-worsening deterioration of health, because biochemical systems do not receive adequate nutrition. People under the age of 35 generally do not require HCL or digestive enzyme supplements, but there are exceptions. If you suffer from gas and bloating or any other signs of incomplete digestion, you may need digestive enzymes. The primary digestive supplements include betaine HCL to supply hydrochloric acid for protein digestion, pancreatin for protein digestion, and bile factors for people who have trouble digesting fat.

The Beyond Vitamins Multisupplement for Youth Extension

For additional information on how to design your personal Beyond Vitamins Program, see Chapter 15.

VITAMINS

Vitamin A	10,000 I.U.
Carotene	25,000 I.U.
Thiamine	50 mg.
Riboflavin	50 mg.
Niacin	50 mg.
Pyridoxine	50 mg.

Pantothenic acid	100 mg.
Folate	400 mcg.
B$_{12}$	100 mcg.
Biotin	400 mcg.
Choline	500 mg. (phosphatidyl, from lecithin)
Inositol	100–250 mg.
Vitamin C	1,000–5,000 mg.
Bioflavonoids	500 mg.
Vitamin E	200–600 I.U.

MINERALS

Calcium	500 mg.
Chromium	100 mcg.
Magnesium	250 mg.
Manganese	10 mg.
Selenium	100 mcg.
Zinc	30–50 mg.

AMINO ACIDS

A good amino acid supplement will contain most of the following amino acids, in varying amounts:

Valine	Leucine
Isoleucine	Glutamine
Phenylalanine	Cystine
Histidine	Methionine
Lysine	Cysteine
Tryptophan	Ornithine
Aspartic acid	Arginine
Glutamic acid	Taurine
Proline	Glycine
Alanine	Tyrosine

AMINO ACIDS FOR INDIVIDUAL USE
(to be taken separately)

Phenylalanine	1,000 mg.
Tyrosine	1,000 mg.
Tryptophan	500–1500 mg.

GLANDULARS

Andrenal	50 mg.
Testicular	50 mg.

GLANDULARS

Ovarian	50 mg.
Pancreas	50 mg.
Thymus	50 mg.
Thyroid	50 mg.
Stomach	50 mg.
Duodenum	50 mg.
Liver	500 mg.
Heart	50 mg.
Pituitary	50 mg.
Brain	50 mg.
Spleen	50 mg.

ENZYMES

Betaine HCL	100 mg.
Pancreatin	100 mg.
Papain	100 mg.
Bromelain	100 mg.
Bile factors	100 mg.

OTHERS

EPA	500 mg.
Mucopolysaccharides	200 mg.

7 Maintaining Maximum Physical and Mental Performance

WE DEMAND a lot from our bodies and minds these days. Peak performance is at the top of most everyone's "Got to Do" list. And even people who've never laced up running shoes or swung a tennis racket find themselves needing that extra 10 to 20 percent of effective effort. Supplements can help you get that extra performance.

In this chapter, we're going to tell you about nutrients that are especially important to stimulating and maintaining maximum mental and physical performance. These supplements will help, whether your major form of exercise is walking or competing in triathalons.

THE BRAIN IS PART OF THE BODY TOO

Maximum performance depends on many factors. For the sake of description and organization, we tend to separate performance into physical and mental. We say that physical performance depends on the muscles, the circulatory system, the pancreas, the adrenal glands—and that mental performance depends on the brain.

But, in reality, they are both part of the same system. You cannot have optimum physical performance without optimum mental performance, and vice versa.

Once again, this is not to say that in order to think at

your best you need to be a world class athlete. Not at all. What we mean is that you must acknowledge that the physical performance does not depend solely on the muscles, and that mental performance does not depend solely on the brain.

In our society, however, we tend to forget that the brain is part of the body. We separate physical and mental, as if the nervous system lived a different life, on a different plane than the other organs and glands. The brain is a physical organ, just like the heart and the liver. Biochemical reactions take place in the brain that are affected by the same factors as those that affect the strength of our muscles and the efficiency of our digestion. Many of these factors are nutritional.

Assuming that the brain is somehow immune to physical factors is only half of the error. The other half is the assumption that the physical body is separate and immune from what the brain does, that the functioning of our organs and glands is not affected by our thoughts and feelings. We know that this is not true. What we think and feel affects our strength and performance just as much as our physical fitness affects our mental functions. The following case illustrates this.

When Neil first walked into my office, I (MR) thought he might be an actor or a model. His wavy, light brown hair and youthful, swarthy good looks did not reveal his forty-two years—or the fact that he was, in fact, an advertising executive. His problem was that he lacked the energy, the motivation, and the will to succeed. Although the first 15 years or so of his career had been wonderful, the last five had been a "living hell." His performance had slowly slipped off, until he had almost been fired from his original firm. "They made it possible for me to resign," he confessed, "and strongly advised me to do so."

After that, Neil worked for three different advertising firms. Two had fired him, and the third had, again, "strongly advised me to resign." Because Neil had designed several extremely successful advertising campaigns early in his career, he was always able to get a job. Someone was always willing to take a chance on him. But he knew those chances were running out.

Understandably, Neil's confidence was just about shot. He complained of insomnia and fretful sleep. He regularly woke up at 4 A.M. His sex drive was very low. Though he had always planned to give up his bachelorhood by age 40, he no longer held out any hope of ever getting married.

Neil had been in in psychotherapy for two years, without much success. He had tried antidepressant drugs, with partial success. But he could not tolerate the side effects, which in his case included dry mouth, constipation, rapid heartbeat, and sedation. So he kept lowering his dose until the drug was ineffective. Finally, he stopped taking the drug and left psychotherapy.

Neil seemed to take reasonable care of himself in most areas. His diet, although deficient because his appetite was low, did not contain any junk food. I advised Neil to take a basic multivitamin-mineral supplement and to try to eat more protein. I suggested that he make himself a salad at least three times a week, and that he consider this activity as recreation, not "cooking."

I decided to try the amino acid tyrosine to boost Neil's moods. He started at a low dose of 500 mg. per day and over the course of a month worked his way up to 3,000 mg. per day (1,000 mg. three times a day). Over a two-month period, Neil gradually improved. He felt more energetic and his attitude grew more positive and confident. His appetites grew stronger too. Although his sleep was still disturbed once a week or so, most of the time he slept through the night and awoke refreshed and ready to start the day.

When Neil reported that he was making salads only twice a week because his ladyfriend was making them, I told him he could lower his dose of tyrosine to 2,000 mg.

I get calls from Neil every now and then. He finally started his own ad agency, in partnership with his new wife.

VITAMINS AND MINERALS TO BOOST PERFORMANCE

Vitamin A supports energy production in many ways. The adrenal glands, which regulate the amount of blood sugar available for energy, require adequate vitamin A. The red blood cells also require vitamin A. The first sign of vitamin A deficiency may, in some persons, be anemia or fatigue. The vitamin A precursor, beta-carotene, is a potent antioxidant. Antioxidants are required in extra amounts by athletes because training levels of activity boost oxygen turnover and create increased amounts of free radicals.

The B vitamins are absolutely essential for maximum performance. Increased demands on all physical and mental systems boost our requirements for the B vitamins, whose primary function is the release of energy from food. The digestive process cannot take place without adequate levels of B vitamins. The adrenal glands, which govern energy output, and the liver, which is part of the body's storehouse of energy, also depend on the B vitamins. Finally, the nervous system cannot coordinate muscular activity without adequate levels of B vitamins. Because the B vitamins are water-soluble, we don't store them for very long and we use them up and excrete them faster under physical and mental stress.

B_1, or thiamine, is a vital coenzyme in the process in which carbohydrates are turned into blood sugar and burned in the cell as fuel for energy. Sweets in the diet raise the requirement for thiamine by temporarily intensifying the "energy flame" and putting a heavier load on the body's regulatory system.

B_2, or riboflavin, is necessary for the cells to "breathe." When riboflavin is inadequately supplied, the cells don't get enough oxygen to produce energy.

B_3, or niacin, is a key nutrient for energy metabolism and mental functioning. Whereas riboflavin is required to enable the cell to use oxygen, niacin is required for the cell to use all major nutrients. Digestive and mental function break down when there is not enough niacin. Niacin supplements have been used successfully to treat some forms of mental illness, aggressive behavior, temper tantrums, restlessness, depression, hyperactivity, and sleep disturbances.

PANTOTHENIC ACID AND THE FAMOUS SWIMMING RATS

Pantothenic acid is the B vitamin most vital to the adrenal glands. Pantothenic acid not only aids in the burning of blood sugar for energy, but also helps the body synthesize and make the most out of the adrenal hormones. By "sparing" adrenal hormones, pantothenic acid prevents the adrenal glands from becoming fatigued. In a classic experiment with swimming rats, it was demonstrated how supplementary amounts of this vitamin can boost performance. One group of rats was given a diet free of pantothenic acid. A second group was given the RDA amount. A third group received supplementary amounts. The deficient rats were able to swim in cold water for only 16 minutes, whereas the RDA rats stayed afloat for 29 minutes. But the supplemented rats swam for 62 minutes.

Two more groups of rats went swimming, both of which had their adrenal glands removed. One group received the RDA amount of pantothenic acid, and the other group received supplementary amounts. The supplemented group not only swam twice as long as the RDA rats with no adrenal glands, but also significantly longer than the first RDA group of rats who still had their adrenals intact!

Later experiments with humans—all with intact adrenal glands!—also demonstrated how pantothenic acid can boost our energy when we need it most. Pantothenic acid is crucial to any supplement program designed to support or improve performance.

B_6, or pyridoxine, also supports performance by its role in the metabolism of carbohydrates, fats, and protein.

Folic acid is required by the red blood cells and the nervous system. Because of the widespread use of antibiotics, which kill intestinal bacteria that manufacture folic acid, and the laws minimizing the amounts of folic acid that can be put in supplements, this vitamin is widely undersupplied. Folic acid deficiency causes a specific type of anemia, the first symptom of which is often weakness.

B_{12} deficiency also causes anemia, weakness, and deterioration of the nervous system. B_{12} deficiency is more likely to occur if you have serious digestive problems, such as gas and bloating. If you're not making enough digestive enzymes, you may not be getting all the B_{12} you need.

Biotin is directly required for carbohydrate metabolism and energy production, and for the support of the thyroid gland and the adrenals.

Choline supports the brain, nervous system, and liver. Choline is a precursor of the neurotransmitter acetylcholine. Supplementary amounts of this vitamin, in the form of phosphatidyl choline derived from lecithin, can boost memory and brain function.

Inositol maintains the capacity of the nerves to conduct impulses. In high doses, inositol can act as a sedative.

VITAMIN C FOR BRAINIER BRAINS AND BRAWNIER BRAWN

Vitamin C boosts both mental and physical functioning. As an antioxidant, vitamin C protects the cells from oxidation during the rapid turnover of oxygen. It also maintains the adrenal glands and muscles, and stimulates the production of adrenal hormones. Exertion and stress mobilize vitamin C and drive up the body's requirement. When the muscles are stressed, their use of vitamin C intensifies, so it makes sense that weakness and fatigue are the early signs of a vitamin C deficiency. Vitamin C supplements can improve alertness, concentration, and other mental functions by stimulating brain pathways that increase catecholamines.

Vitamin E's value to performance lies in its ability to maximize oxygen utilization and protect the cells from oxidation.

BIOFLAVONOIDS BOOST PERFORMANCE

By strengthening the tissues, reducing inflammation, serving as an antioxidant, and boosting the effectiveness of vitamin C, bioflavonoids earn a major role in the Beyond Vitamins Multisupplement for Maximum Performance.

Inflammation can be the enemy of performance. When tissues swell and become painful, you can't perform or train at a normal pace. Here's how bioflavonoids will help you reduce inflammation. The cement substance that holds the walls of the membranes and blood vessels together is thickened by bioflavonoids, so they become less fragile and likely to leak. So when there is an injury, inflammation is reduced because the amount of tissue damage and leaking of blood and fluids into the area is minimized.

BIOFLAVONOIDS ALSO DEACTIVATE INFLAMMATION AT THE SOURCE

Bioflavonoids also reduce inflammation by deactivating enzymes that produce inflammatory prostaglandins. Quercetin, a form of the bioflavonoid rutin, shows great promise as an anti-inflammatory supplement that can reduce asthma and other allergy-type reactions. This bioflavonoid apparently prevents the mast cells from discharging histamine and other inflammatory substances.

BIOFLAVONOIDS SPEED HEALING

By strengthening the tiny blood vessels, which tend to rupture, and by reducing inflammation, bioflavonoids also speed healing from athletic sprains, strains, and other injuries.

HIGH PERFORMANCE MINERALS

Calcium is important to performance for many reasons. Each time you do some kind of weight-bearing exercise, which includes just about everything except swimming, bone metabolism increases. That means calcium turnover from the bones to the blood, and back again to the bones, is stepped up. It's inevitable that some of the calcium turned over into the bloodstream is going to be excreted. Normally, exercise causes the bones to retain more calcium and grow in strength, but if dietary calcium is inadequate, the bones may suffer a net loss in calcium.

Muscle and nerve excitability are also regulated by calcium in the blood and tissues. When calcium levels are inadequate, the muscles and nerves become more irritable, which makes them tire more easily.

Chromium, the active principle in glucose tolerance factor, is vital to energy production. Chromium is a cofactor with insulin. Without adequate chromium, insulin is less effective in stimulating the uptake of blood sugar into the cells. Fatigue, irritability, depression, and other symptoms of impaired sugar tolerance may result when chromium is not supplied. Stress, exercise, infection, trauma, and a high-sugar diet use up chromium at a faster rate. Runners, for example, excrete twice as much chromium on days that they run as on days when they are idle.

Iodine is required for the function of the thyroid gland. Trace amounts of this mineral present in multimineral supplements of iodized salt and salt substitutes should provide enough. If you are on a low- or no-salt diet, you should check to make sure your diet contains some source of this vital mineral.

Iron is required for adequate energy production, because the red blood cells need it in order to deliver oxygen to the cells. The only people who require regular iron supplements, however, are pregnant, nursing, or menstruating women, or people who suffer injury, blood loss, or malnutrition.

Magnesium stimulates performance through its effects on the muscles and nerves. Not only does this mineral boost respiration, but, when teamed up with potassium, it can increase energy, stamina, and endurance. When given to people suffering from chronic fatigue, lassitude, morning fatigue, insomnia, headaches, lower back pain, and other vague pains, a combined magnesium-potassium supplement can relieve symptoms and restore energy.

Potassium regulates the irritability of muscles and nerves and helps determine how soon you become fatigued.

Manganese supports blood sugar regulation by insulin and is also required for the strength of the tendons, ligaments, and vertebral discs. When training or recovering from an injury, you should increase your manganese intake.

Selenium is important as an antioxidant, helping to protect the tissues from oxidant damage.

Zinc is absolutely vital to maximum performance. Zinc supports the pancreas, which regulates the body's use of blood sugar. Zinc is also necessary for muscle growth and regeneration. Performance uses up muscle tissue, and zinc is required to rebuild that lost tissue. When you train, the body is constantly tearing down and rebuilding, and growing in strength while it heals. Zinc is the principal nutrient to stimulate healing and is a necessary part of any training program.

Zinc may also be useful in keeping the mental aspects of performance fully functioning. Zinc deficiency has been shown to be a factor in depression, bulimia, anorexia, and other neurotic states.

AMINO ACID ENERGY FACTORS

Free-form amino acids can help boost your energy. These supplements consist of amino acids, which are manufactured by bacteria in such a way that they are separate, not linked together as they often appear in food. The rationale for using these supplements is that they are very easily absorbed and do not rely on digestion to break them down.

There is some controversy surrounding the use of these combined amino acid supplements. Some claims have been made that these amino acids supply little more than an expensive boost in blood sugar, one that could just as easily be obtained with a dose of sugar. There is some truth to this claim, especially if the amino acids are taken on an empty stomach. They are so rapidly absorbed that they literally flood the liver with amino acids, forcing it to convert a higher percentage of the protein to blood sugar. Arguably, this is a higher-quality energy boost than one you might obtain from a tablespoon of sugar.

To get this boost, you must take from 10 to 15 capsules or tablets at one time, with a little fruit juice to enhance absorption.

INDIVIDUAL AMINO ACIDS
AND PERFORMANCE

Leucine, isoleucine, and valine are known as the "branched-chain" amino acids. All three play major roles in the regulation of blood sugar and energy. The muscles seem to prefer these amino acids and use them for energy production before they use others. These amino acids can boost stamina and endurance, as well as prevent low blood sugar. Leucine also supports the healing of injured skin and bones.

Tryptophan can boost your physical and mental performance by relaxing you and helping you get a good night's sleep. One or two grams of tryptophan taken with some fruit juice or sweetened nonfat milk one-half to one hour before bedtime will help you sleep.

Taken during the day, tryptophan can relieve some forms of depression and act as a natural tranquilizer. Sometimes the only thing holding you back from maximum performance is your own nervous energy. Tryptophan can help relieve that and enable you to direct your energy usefully.

Like tryptophan, glycine and glutamic acid tone down brain function. Glutamic acid forms GABA, or gamma-amino butyric acid, an inhibitory brain neurotransmitter. If you're nervous and tense, you can't perform at peak levels either mentally or physically. These amino acids can help you relax.

Carnitine boosts energy by stimulating the body's burning of fats (tryglycerides, mainly) as fuel. By burning fat as fuel, the body's supply of glycogen stored in the liver is spared for heavier exertion. Generally, the body will burn fat up to 75 to 80 percent of maximum exertion. After that, glycogen from carbohydrates is burned. By burning more fat and saving more glycogen, you not only reduce your fat stores and slim down, but you also increase your stamina and endurance. Regular use of carnitine in high doses (2 to 4 grams per day) can boost your VO_2 max, which is a measure of the body's aerobic capacity. The higher your VO_2 max, the more oxygen your body is able to process to produce energy. Higher VO_2 max means more strength, stamina, and endurance.

Carnitine is not considered an "essential" amino acid because the body does synthesize its own carnitine from the amino acid lysine. There is evidence, however, that we don't always manufacture enough, either for baseline or optimal functioning.

Phenylalanine and tyrosine are antidepressants and stimulants that can boost mental performance. Phenylalanine has the added benefit of helping to reduce the pain and soreness of muscles. Both of these amino acids increase the brain's supply of catecholamines, neurotransmitters that boost mood, self-esteem, energy, reduce sensitivity to aches and pains, relieve anxiety and depression, stimulate ambition and aggression, and generally keep us awake and alert. It is normally not necessary to take both of these amino acids. People with high blood pressure, however, should not take phenylalanine. These amino acids, like tryptophan, should be taken on an empty stomach.

Methionine is also valuable to boost energy. This amino acid is a potent antioxidant and will help vitamins A, C, and E, selenium, and zinc protect the tissues from increased oxidation caused by increased oxygen turnover.

Aspartic acid is another amino acid that boosts excitatory neurotransmitters—particularly those that stimulate sensory perception. Russian cosmonauts have experimented with aspartic acid during space flights, and have found that it improves performance during heavy mental and physical work. You don't have to be in outer space in order to enjoy the benefits of aspartic acid, however.

Lysine, as an essential amino acid, does have officially recognized deficiency symptoms, which include fatigue, reduced concentration, irritability, bloodshot eyes, and anemia. Most people know about lysine through its use as an antiherpes supplement. But the amino acid can also be useful to people whose performance is regularly interrupted by migraine headaches.

Glutamine is known for its ability to reduce the craving for alcohol and sweets, but it is also capable of improving brain function and memory. Glutamine is low in the blood of people with low blood sugar. Glutamine should be taken separately, on an empty stomach. Some people find that taking it with B_6 improves its effectiveness.

Arginine increases muscle tone, boosts pituitary function, stimulates growth hormone release, and increases fat burning—all of which can improve performance. Ornithine, an amino acid that is usually grouped with arginine because both stimulate growth hormone release, has an effect similar to that of GTF chromium: It lowers blood sugar by maximizing the effects of insulin.

ENZYMES FOR FULL DIGESTION AND FULL POWER

If you do not digest your food completely, you will not get the full benefit from the nutrients in the food or in your supplements. How do you know if you're not digesting your food completely? If you have gas, bloating, burping, and belching after you eat, then chances are good you're not fully digesting your food. Gas, bloating, and flatulence result when bacteria in the gut go to work on undigested food particles. If you have these problems, betaine hydrochloride will help raise your hydrochloric acid, and pancreatic enzymes will boost your pancreatin to fully digest proteins, carbohydrates, and fats.

Enzyme supplements should not necessarily be a permanent addition to your life. If you need them, it's an indication that you need to restore full function to your digestive system. Your increased supplementation and a program to manage your food allergies effectively will help you rebuild these organs and glands. (See Chapter 10.)

ENZYMES INSTEAD OF ASPIRIN

When we're injured, the body rushes fluids to the site, fluids that are useful in healing and preventing further injury or infection. Sometimes, however, the swelling and edema are heightened by a slowdown in the body's usual pathways for moving the fluids. The gathering fluids, although initially useful, now become a problem. Chemicals in the fluids cause pain when they press on exposed nerves.

Often, the slowdown in fluids transport is caused by clotting blood or dead tissue blocking the normal paths. Proteolytic, or protein-digesting, enzymes are very effective in reducing pain and swelling after injuries by breaking down dead tissue and blood clots.

As a matter of fact, proteolytic enzymes, in combination with vitamin C and bioflavonoids, can be more effective than aspirin and other nonsteroidal anti-inflammatory drugs, for reducing pain, swelling, edema, and heat of inflammation caused by injury. Trypsin, papain, bromelain, and pancreatin can be used to reduce soreness and speed the healing of bruises resulting from minor athletic injuries. Papain and bromelain have also been used successfully to reduce pain and swelling after oral surgery.

OCTACOSANOL FOR STAMINA

Octacosanol is a complex fatty acid that is concentrated from wheat germ oil. Several studies, as well as clinical experience, demonstrate that this supplement can increase stamina and endurance. It takes at least two months to achieve this effect, however.

GAMMA-LINOLENIC ACID IS ESSENTIAL FOR HIGH PERFORMANCE

In previous chapters, we've described how gamma-linolenic acid (GLA) is required for the body's production of the PG1 series of prostaglandins. These prostaglandins stimulate a wide range of functions, including energy production and mental performance. PG1 prostaglandins boost the effectiveness of insulin. PG1 prostaglandins also play a role in preventing depression and schizophrenia. In people suffering from these disorders, PG1 levels can be low.

EPA CAN KEEP YOUR HEAD CLEAR OF MIGRAINE PAIN

People who do not suffer from migraine headaches often cannot understand how completely debilitating these attacks can be. Although the causes of migraine are not fully understood, there are nontoxic, natural nutritional supplements that can bring some relief and restore functioning. EPA from fish oil is one such supplement. It can reduce the intensity and frequency of migraine attacks, if used daily for more than four to six weeks. A study of the effects of EPA from fish oil on hundreds of migraine sufferers found that the supplement either freed people totally from pain or greatly reduced their pain until they characterized it as "mild."

DMG SPARKS YOUR ENGINE

DMG is a favorite of athletes, especially those from the Soviet Union and eastern European nations. As an antioxidant, DMG helps spare oxygen and prevent oxidative damage to the tissues during the rapid oxygen turnover of exercise. It helps the cells get by with less oxygen, a boon to all of us, not just athletes.

But DMG does more than that; it improves mental and physical performance in many ways. DMG increases blood sugar, boosts oxygen utilization, and reduces fatigue-causing lactate levels in the muscles. As a result, energy and strength are increased, whereas fatigue and soreness are decreased. The time it takes you to become exhausted become greater and the capacity of your body to process oxygen—VO$_2$ max—is boosted. By how much? Well, in one study of DMG's effects on athletic performance, supplementation over the course of a week increased treadmill running time by 24 percent and boosted VO$_2$ max by 27 percent.

From other experiments, we know that DMG stimulates adrenal function, and it supports cardiovascular function by normalizing heart rhythm and increasing the heart muscle's uptake and utilization of oxygen. DMG also supports the liver's metabolism of fat, lowers cholesterol, and normalizes sugar metabolism.

DMG also improves mental functioning by increasing the supply of oxygen to the brain. This is, of course, valuable to those of us who want to boost our already-normal functioning to optimal levels. But it is of even greater value to the mentally retarded persons in whom DMG has been able to lessen the frequency of seizures.

GLANDULARS TO REGENERATE ENERGY

Adrenal substance may be a very important glandular supplement for maintaining and increasing your energy supply. The adrenal glands are responsible for stimulating and regulating the body's energy metabolism. In response to stress or a challenge, the adrenal hormones stimulate energy production through an increase in heart rate and respiration, dilation of blood vessels, and increase in blood sugar.

Pancreas substance can help boost performance by stimulating endocrine function controlling the utilization of blood sugar and supporting digestion. The pancreas has two roles. The first is to secrete insulin to regulate the uptake of blood sugar by the cells. The second is to secrete the digestive enzyme pancreatin, which digests carbohydrates, fats, and protein. Pancreas substance is also very high in picolinates, substances that greatly enhance the absorption of zinc.

Liver is an important supplement for performance. Liver is so rich in natural energy-boosting nutrients that it's a must for any supplement program designed to maximize health and performance. We know that liver is high in vitamins, minerals, nucleic acids, and amino acids. Liver is an especially good source of GTF-chromium, the mineral that increases energy by raising the effectiveness of insulin.

But there are, no doubt, other, as yet undiscovered, factors in liver that boost performance. Raw liver concentrate was actually one of the first supplements. In classic animal experiments, liver boosted strength, endurance, performance, and resistance to stress and disease. The effect was not due to any known vitamins or minerals in the liver. The "control" group of animals that did not receive liver were given supplements of all the known vitamins and minerals contained in liver. Still, their performance did not come close to that of the liver-supplemented animals.

Heart substance is also a good glandular supplement for performance. The heart muscle, after all, is the pump that keeps the entire body machine moving.

AND DON'T FORGET
THESE IMPORTANT ENERGY FACTS

No matter how many supplements you take, you still must eat a diet that will also support mental and physical performance. Performance requires energy, and energy is supplied by the burning of blood sugar by the cells. Blood sugar is derived from food. By far the best sources of energy in the diet are complex carbohydrates. Refined carbohydrates and sugars are digested and absorbed too fast, resulting in a strain on the enzyme and glandular systems that regulate energy. After an initial quick boost in energy, the body can slump back. Complex carbohydrates are digested more slowly; they release blood sugar into the system at a rate the body can comfortably handle.

It's also a good idea to eat some high quality protein with

your carbohydrates. Protein in the meal will stimulate the secretions of hydrochloric acid and digestive enzymes, which will enable you to get the most out of all your food.

WATER IS AN ABSOLUTE NECESSITY FOR MAXIMUM PERFORMANCE

One last nutrient, and one of supreme importance—water. No matter how much of the best foods you eat, no matter how many supplements you take, you'll be exhausted and feel miserable if you don't drink enough water. We're convinced that dehydration is a very widespread, unrecognized problem. Dehydration drains your energy, gives you a headache, and fuzzes your brain. Performing—whether you're doing it at a desk, on a stage, or on an athletic field—will use up water. All of the body's metabolic business requires water, including digestion.

The myth that it's not a good idea to drink water with meals is just that—a myth. Drinking water with a meal does not dilute digestive enzymes or hydrochloric acid; it gives them a medium for dissolving and digesting the food. So sip water during your meal and then take your supplements with a glass of water after your meal. Drink water between meals, and when you're going to be exercising, sweating, or exerting yourself in any way. Drink extra water before you feel thirsty, because thirst is a sign that it's too late, you're already compromising your body's ability to perform mentally and physically at peak levels.

Here's an example of how Beyond Vitamins supplements can help.

Mary and John had met at the San Francisco Bay-to-Breakers Footrace, a wild, festive jogging free-for-all in which tens of thousands of people dress up in every conceivable way and run from San Francisco Bay on one side of the city to the Pacific Ocean on the other side. John was in costume as a "human jukebox," and Mary ran as the last set of legs in a 12-woman "cable car centipede."

After their marriage, they continued to jog together. They often combined vacations in exotic locales, such as Hawaii and New Zealand, with marathons and other road races.

John and Mary were not my patients. We met at a mutual friend's birthday party. I (MR) noticed they were both taking it easy on their feet, almost limping. Other than that, they appeared to be healthy, vigorous thirty-five year-olds. I asked them why they were limping.

Both of them had sore legs. They had been in training for a race and their muscles, tendons, ligaments, and joints were, as Mary put it, "responding in the usual way." In other words, they expected to feel this way after running.

I asked them about their training habits, and it appeared that they were careful to stretch and rest their legs at the appropriate times. And they really didn't push themselves too hard. To them, running in these races was a celebration, not a competition. They sometimes walked several miles, and even when they ran, they never pushed themselves too hard.

Actually, John and Mary weren't complaining at all!

I asked them what supplements they took.

Mary said that she took a basic miltivitamin-mineral supplement. John said he wasn't taking any supplements, although he had taken an "athletic stress formula" for several years but had stopped after he read in a running magazine that supplements weren't necessary. I asked John if he remembered what was in the supplement. He recalled that it had about 250 mg. of vitamin C and 25 mg. of the B vitamins. "That's all?" I asked.

"That's all, he replied.

"If you don't mind my saying, that's not nearly enough —and it's not all the things every person who exercises as much as you two needs."

I went on to explain to John and Mary that their exercising greatly increased their requirements for certain nutrients, and that their sore legs might be relieved if they took better care of their nutritional status.

They asked for specifics, so I told them about the supplements described in this chapter. They wrote them down.

I didn't see John and Mary again until a year later, at the same friend's house. This time they didn't appear to be nursing sore limbs. I was tempted to ask them if they were still running, or if they'd started taking supplements, but I didn't have to ask. They saw me, came over, and told me themselves.

They had started taking the supplements I had recommended. At first, they were skeptical. Not very much changed for more than three months. Then, Mary noticed something. Their hot water bill went down—even though the rates had gone up! What does this have to do with supplements?

After their daily runs together, they took a shower together. They used the hot shower to help relax their muscles so they could stretch them out and relieve some of the soreness. Sometimes they also filled the bathtub with hot water and soaked their legs. Well, apparently, those showers were getting shorter. Their legs were less sore than before.

Mary and John became believers. They increased their doses of the anti-inflammatory nutrients and, after a few weeks, noticed that their soreness was reduced even further. And when they had flare-ups, the supplements helped them heal faster.

And they saved money on their hot water bill.

The Beyond Vitamins Multisupplement for Maximum Performance

For additional information on how to design your personal Beyond Vitamins Program, see Chapter 15.
*(M) = With Meals (B) = Between Meals (N) = At Night
(BB) = Before Breakfast

VITAMINS

Vitamin A	10,000 I.U.
Carotene	25,000–50,000 I.U.

Thiamine	100 mg.
Riboflavin	100 mg.
Niacin	100–500 mg.
Pyridoxine	100 mg.
Pantothenic Acid	100–500 mg.
Folate	400 mcg.
B$_{12}$	100 mcg.
Biotin	400 mcg.
Choline	1,000–10,000 mg. (phosphatidyl)
Inositol	100 mg.
PABA	100 mg.
Vitamin C	4,000–8,000 mg.
Bioflavonoids	500–2,000 mg.
Vitamin E	400–800 I.U.

MINERALS

Calcium	500 mg.
Chromium	200–500 mcg.
Iodine	100 mcg.
Magnesium	250 mg.
Manganese	10–15 mg.
Potassium	100–200 mg.
Selenium	200 mcg.
Zinc	30 mg.

FREE FORM AMINO ACIDS

A good amino acid supplement will contain most of the following amino acids, in varying amounts:

Valine	Leucine
Isoleucine	Glutamine
Phenylalanine	Cystine
Histidine	Methionine
Lysine	Cysteine
Tryptophan	Ornithine
Aspartic acid	Arginine
Glutamic acid	Taurine
Proline	Glycine
Alanine	Tyrosine

INDIVIDUAL AMINO ACIDS
(to be taken for specific purposes)

Carnitine	500–5,000 mg. (M)*
Methionine	100–500 mg. (M)

INDIVIDUAL AMINO ACIDS
(to be taken for specific purposes)

Glutathione	100–500 mg. (M)
Isoleucine	100–1,000 mg. (M)
Valine	100–1,000 mg. (M)
Leucine	100–1,000 mg. (M)
Glycine	100–1,000 mg. (M)
Tyrosine	500–2,000 mg. (B)*
Glutamic acid	100–1,000 mg. (M)
Tryptophan	500–2,000 mg. (N)* or (BB)*
Lysine	500–3,000 mg. (M)
Aspartic acid	5–1,000 mg. (M)
Phenylalanine	500–2,000 mg. (B)
Arginine	500–1,000 mg. (M)
Ornithine	500–1,000 mg. (M)

GLANDULARS

Adrenal	50 mg.
Pancreas	50 mg.
Liver	500 mg.
Heart	50 mg.

ENZYMES

Betaine HCL	100 mg.
Pancreatin	100 mg.
Papain	100–500 mg.
Bromelain	100–500 mg.

OTHERS

EPA	500–1,000 mg.
Octacosanol	250 mcg.
Mucopolysaccharides	200 mg.
DMG	100–200 mg.

CHAPTER

8 Nutrition Secrets to Help You Lose Weight —on Any Diet!

ABOUT TWO-THIRDS of the adults in this country are either on a diet or believe they should be. Dieting to lose weight is a way of life for most Americans.

Our aim here is not to prescribe the perfect diet. We aim, instead, to give some recommendations for nutrients that will help any diet do the job faster and better. We're going to assume some common goals for all diets, then talk about supplements that may help you achieve those specific goals.

We assume, first of all, that the principal goal of a diet is to lose weight. Achieving that goal is not difficult, theoretically. It's the magic of actually making it happen—and making it stay happened—that is full of mystery.

Hence the secondary goal of a diet: to somehow manipulate physics and biology so that the first goal is not only possible, but easy.

A lot of things get in the way. And every new diet that's invented promises to remove those obstacles in a new and entertaining way. Here is our contribution to making your diet more effective and lasting. We will recommend supplements that can help you:

- Increase the efficiency of digestion
- Promote the metabolism of fat, carbohydrates, and protein
- Stimulate energy
- Reduce cravings
- Suppress the appetite and calm the nerves

INCREASE DIGESTIVE EFFICIENCY

This may, at first, seem contradictory. Don't you want to decrease digestion so that less food is absorbed? No, because one of the major causes of overeating is poor nutrition. The body knows what it needs and it tries its best to get it. When we don't get all the nutrients we need, the body's deep, silent hunger for better nutrition is expressed in our own desire for more food.

You don't have to be a junk food junkie in order to be a victim of malnutrition. As we've pointed out earlier, you might be eating a good diet and taking supplements, but still not absorbing the nutrients you think you are. This state of affairs can make you desire to eat more. Your body will express its hunger for better food as a hunger for more food.

Well, you might ask, if my digestion isn't working so well, why do I put on weight?

This is a good question. The answer is that carbohydrates are the easiest food to digest, insofar as the starch or sugar components are easier to separate, break down, and absorb. Protein is harder to digest and absorb, and poor digestion often results in protein deficiencies. Fat is the most difficult, but there's so much fat in most American diets that there's always plenty to absorb. And getting all your vitamins and minerals is almost as difficult as getting all your protein.

If you increase the efficiency of your digestion while on a diet—or any other time for that matter—you will absorb more nutrients and be more satisfied.

To boost your digestive efficiency, you need digestive enzymes, especially pancreatin, which will increase the efficiency of protein digestion. Betaine hydrochloride will also enhance protein digestion because it adds to the hydrochloric acid in your stomach and also stimulates the secretion of natural digestive enzymes. Bile factors will help you digest fat.

To further support the strength of your digestive glands and organs, these glandular supplements may help: pancreas substance, stomach substance, and duodenum substance.

PROMOTE FAT, CARBOHYDRATE, AND PROTEIN METABOLISM

Once you've made your digestive system more efficient and increased your absorption of nutrients, you also want to increase the body's efficiency in using these nutrients. In the case of fat, you want to promote the burning of fat for fuel, for obvious reasons. If your body doesn't handle the fat gingerly, so to speak, it's more likely to wind up in your liver or around your middle. Also, when your intake of fat, protein, and carbohydrates is reduced, the body is going to have to metabolize fat out of storage for energy.

Most people take for granted that the body is just going to burn fat for fuel whenever it needs to. It's not as simple as that. The biochemical operation that burns fat for fuel requires several metabolic steps, all of which need the right cofactors to be there at the right time. The nutrients that are important cofactors in the process of metabolizing fat properly are carnitine, methionine, taurine, vitamin A, choline, inositol, folic acid, pyridoxine, B_{12}, and DMG.

CARNITINE MAY BE THE DIETER'S DREAM COME TRUE

Carnitine is the nonessential amino acid that may prove to be indispensable to people who want to lose weight. Carnitine's value to dieters lies in its ability to stimulate the body's burning of fat for energy. Carnitine is officially classified as nonessential, because the body manufactures it from the essential amino acids lysine and methionine (in the presence of adequate vitamin C). There is evidence, however, that we don't always manufacture all the carnitine that we need. And there is also plenty of evidence that supplying extra carnitine can help boost the body's clearance of fat. By making more fat available to the muscles, carnitine also increases our energy supply.

Carnitine has been used as a supplement primarily to boost energy and stamina for athletes and to lower blood levels of fat and invigorate the heart muscle in people with cardiovascular disease. Its use as a dieter's aid has only begun to be developed.

LIVER ALSO BOOSTS FAT CLEARANCE

Liver substance should also be a part of any supplement program to promote fat metabolism, because the liver is the principal site of fat metabolism. Liver concentrate supplements will also boost energy production through enhancement of sugar metabolism.

Proper metabolism of protein and carbohydrates is also desirable while you're on a diet, especially a high-protein diet. Such diets can strain the body's ability to squeeze energy out of available food. Remember, the body is not 100 percent efficient in making up the difference between the energy it needs and the energy it gets in the diet. You have to give it all the help you can.

The B vitamins are the major supporters of protein and carbohydrate metabolism. Calcium is also a good idea if you're on a high-protein diet. Such diets cause increased requirements for calcium.

GLA ALSO STOKES THE BODY'S FAT FURNACE

Some of the most interesting new evidence about how the body burns fat for energy revolves around the issue of brown fat, which is believed to be the most metabolically active fat in the body, as opposed to white fat, which is less active. Theoretically, people who have trouble staying thin have less brown fat than others. It may also be true, however, that such people have brown fat, which is less metabolically active.

Whichever theory is true, the point is that if we can boost the metabolic activity of whatever brown fat we have, the body will burn up its fat stores more quickly. Fortunately, there is more than theory to help us out here—there's gamma-linolenic acid. GLA has been shown to stimulate the brown fat and boost the body's use of its fat stores.

Every overweight person has steadfastly held on to the conviction that thin people stay slim not because they eat less, but because of some metabolic secret that thin bodies contain which theirs do not. As science confirms what we overweight people knew all along, thankfully we're also coming up with ways (e.g., the use of carnitine and GLA) to shift the metabolic odds closer to being, if not in our favor, at least closer to even.

CAN YOU FIRE UP YOUR BODY'S FURNACE WITH THYROID SUBSTANCE?

How about boosting the metabolism with thyroid glandulars? We don't think it's a particularly good idea when you're on a diet, because the supplement may increase hormone production. Excess thyroid hormone stimulates the wasting of muscle tissue, not fat tissue. Of course, if your diet is adequate in all nutrients, or if you have a thyroid deficiency, then thyroid hormone will not have this effect. But for someone on a diet, and who is probably in negative balance for protein, you want to do everything you can to preserve muscle tissue.

STIMULATE ENERGY WHILE DIETING

One of the major complaints of people on diets is that they have no energy. Increased digestive and metabolic efficiency will go a long way toward improving energy. However, there are still some supplements you can try.

Vitamin C and the B vitamins, especially pantothenic acid, and adrenal substance will support the adrenal glands, which regulate the body's energy supply.

Potassium and magnesium will increase energy and improve sleep.

Manganese and chromium will boost energy production by improving blood sugar metabolism.

Octocosanol will, over the course of several weeks, improve stamina and endurance, of which you may need all you can get when you're on a diet.

Leucine, isoleucine, and valine, the branched-chain amino acids, are valuable to maintaining energy while dieting. Free-form amino acids may also be of value, not only as a source of quick energy but also to improve protein balance. When we eat fewer calories than we need, we do not always get all the protein we require. Thus the body is often forced to metabolize protein for energy.

YOU CAN REDUCE THOSE CRAVINGS

Cravings usually result from food allergies. Chapter 10 contains a complete discussion of supplements for reducing food allergies.

The amino acid glutamine can help you reduce cravings for sweets and alcohol.

SUPPRESS YOUR APPETITE

Most of the drive to eat comes not from the stomach but from the nervous system, and it usually results not from a lack of food in the gut but from an imbalance of nervous impulses in the brain. Whether those impulses come from early childhood experiences, food allergies, or purely chemical factors, we are often driven to eat in order to soothe them. Most overeating is simply compulsive, driven, thoughtless eating. Suppression of appetite, then, should focus on the brain.

The amino acids phenylalanine and tryptophan are useful for relaxation, antidepression, and appetite suppression. Tryptophan supplements tend to diminish the desire for carbohydrates, but this can be a double-edged sword for dieters. It's true that many overweight people have gotten that way because they have sought out carbohydrate foods. It's also true, however, that complex carbohydrate foods are among the best foods dieters can eat. Complex carbohydrates (e.g., whole grains and potatoes) are digested at a slower rate than simple carbohydrates (sugars, sweets, refined flours), so they release blood sugar into the system at a slower rate, thus keeping energy high and hunger low for longer periods.

Of course, many overweight people do not satisfy their desire for carbohydrates with complex carbohydrates. They favor sweet, processed carbohydrate snack foods. Still, although complex carbohydrates such as spaghetti no longer deserve to be called "fattening," they do need to be controlled in many diets. Tryptophan and glutamine (which reduces the craving for sweets) should help do that. After all, they don't destroy the desire for carbohydrates, they simply diminish it.

Many dieters suffer from insomnia. Tryptophan can also

help them: 500 to 1,500 mg. taken one hour before bedtime with a half glass of milk sweetened with honey or fruit juice will help induce relaxation and sleep.

Phenylalanine suppresses the appetite by stimulating the neurotransmitters in the brain that control all of our appetites and drives. In other words, phenylalanine works by stimulating our other appetites and desires, while diminishing the one for food. Many overweight people overeat because they're depressed. Phenylalanine boosts the antidepressant neurotransmitters and helps relieve depression.

VITAMINS AND MINERALS THAT HELP BALANCE MOODS

The B vitamins are also useful in balancing hormones and neurotransmitters that affect moods. Magnesium and calcium are muscle relaxants that can calm the nerves and soothe the muscles.

THE SIMPLEST, CHEAPEST WEIGHT-LOSS SUPPLEMENTS

Finally, two nutrients that are quite valuable to dieters are bran (or fiber) and water. Fiber provides bulk and improves digestion and elimination. Fiber also removes fat from the body, lowers cholesterol, and slows sugar absorption. When sugar absorption is too rapid, insulin levels rise, resulting in more fat deposition and a quicker return to hunger. Without adequate water in the diet, however, extra fiber can actually cause constipation. You should drink a glass of water for every tablespoon of extra bran in your diet. (You can soak the bran before eating it, or cook it in water, as you would oatmeal.) Water also aids in digestion, provides a medium for metabolic reactions to take place, and helps eliminate toxic by-products of weight loss.

Here is a case where Beyond Vitamins supplements helped a dieter to succeed: Kimberly, a thirty-four-year-old executive in the San Francisco city government, was 5 feet 4 inches, and weighed 180 pounds. Her ideal weight should have been about 125 pounds, but she had been overweight since she was eighteen. Before she came to see me (MR), she had been on several diets. She could lose weight gradually on a diet, but she always reached a point beyond which she could not lose any more. At that point she always got discouraged and gained back all the weight she had lost. She had not gone below 145 pounds for more than 10 years.

Kimberly was, by her own admission, a victim of compulsive eating—mainly of sweets and breads. If she ate any bread or anything sweet, she could not stop. Except for her compulsive eating of sweets, her general diet was fine. I suspected that her cravings might come from food allergies, so I tested her.

Sure enough, Kimberly was allergic to sugar, wheat, and baker's yeast. I instructed her to eliminate these foods for 90 days, with the promise that at some point she would probably be able to eat them again, but in moderate quantities. I explained to her that once she "got them out of her system" by eliminating them totally, she would not be so easily drawn into the cycle of cravings and compulsive eating. To replace the lost cereal fiber, I recommended oat bran.

To help Kimberly deal with her cravings, I also told her to take, in addition to a basic multivitamin-mineral supplement, some chromium (200 mcg. at each meal) to help make her body's utilization of sugar more efficient. This usually reduces the body's craving for more sugar. Also, she was instructed to take phenylalanine (500 mg. three times a day) to suppress her appetite and raise her moods; and glutamine (500 mg. three times a day) to further reduce her craving for sweets.

I advised Kimberly to take a general amino acid formula

that contained the branched chain amino acids (leucine, isoleucine, and valine) to help increase her energy levels, and alanine to help her maintain normal blood sugar levels. Finally, I told her to take some carnitine (500 mg. twice a day) to help her body break down fat and burn it for energy.

Kimberly did well on her diet. In the first month she lost 15 pounds, and was amazed that, unlike any of her previous diets, she actually had more energy than when she was eating everything in sight! For the first two weeks she did have some withdrawal cravings for sweets and wheat bread. But her supplements helped her glide over those periods.

During the second month, she lost another 12 pounds, and she was ecstatic! She reported that she didn't miss sugar or wheat products at all.

The third month was when the moment of truth arrived. Kimberly was now approaching the weight below which she had not dropped in over a decade. She confessed to some anxiety, but said she felt confident that she could do it.

And she did. During the last week of the third month, Kimberly sailed below 145 pounds and kept right on going. She finished off the month at 142.

She now had the option of slowly returning wheat products to her diet, on a limited basis, of course. But Kimberly decided she wanted to get below 130 pounds before she tried that. She said she felt no desire to eat wheat or sweets anyway. I supported her decision. In the coming months she lost another 16 pounds. She was able to reduce her extra Beyond Vitamins supplements. And she is free of her cravings. Every now and then she will have some fresh bread and even a dessert if the occasion is special. But she never eats compulsively and her weight fluctuates between 127 and 130.

The Beyond Vitamins Multisupplement for Weight Loss

For additional information on how to design your personal
Beyond Vitamins Program, see Chapter 15

VITAMINS

Vitamin A	10,000 I.U.
Thiamine	50 mg.
Riboflavin	50 mg.
Niacin	50 mg.
Pyridoxine	50 mg.
Pantothenic Acid	100 mg.
Folate	400 mcg.
B_{12}	100 mcg.
Biotin	400 mcg.
Choline	250 mg.
Inositol	100 mg.
PABA	100 mg.
Vitamin C	1,000–4,000 mg.
Bioflavonoids	200–1,000 mg.
Vitamin E	100–400 I.U.

MINERALS

Calcium	500–1,000 mg.
Chromium	200 mcg.
Magnesium	250–500 mg.
Manganese	10 mg.
Potassium	100 mg.

AMINO ACIDS

Glutamine	100–1,000 mg.
Carnitine	500–4,000 mg.
Cystine	100 mg.
Methionine	100 mg.
Glutathione	100–250 mg.
Leucine	100–500 mg.
Isoleucine	100–500 mg.
Valine	100–500 mg.
Taurine	100–500 mg.
Tryptophan	500–1,500 mg. (separately)
Phenylalanine	500–1,000 mg. (separately)

GLANDULARS

Adrenal	50 mg.
Pancreas	50 mg.
Stomach	50 mg.
Duodenum	50 mg.
Liver	500 mg.

ENZYMES

Betaine HCL	100 mg.
Pancreatin	100 mg.
Bile Factors	100 mg.

OTHERS

Octacosanol	250 mcg.
DMG	100–200 mg.
GLA	50–250 mg. (500–2,500 EPO)

9 Supplements *Can* Improve Your Sex Life

WE HUMANS ARE, in a word, insatiable. It's human always to want more.

It's also human to be different and have different needs and appetites. Just as our nutritional requirements differ from individual to individual, so does the sexual appetite. What's too much for some people is not enough for others. Also, different situations and physiological circumstances will have varying effects on sexual desire and potency.

SEXUAL POWER IS OFTEN THE FIRST VICTIM OF MALNUTRITION

Because good sex depends on the functioning of so many parts of the body, it's often the first to be affected when our health becomes imbalanced. The body can just lose the desire and the ability to reproduce when it is not healthy. Sexual desire can disappear with viral and other infections, during periods of intense hunger, and in many diseases. But you don't have to be down and out sick to have your sexual desire and performance affected. Some fairly healthy people can have sexual difficulties.

Sex, after all, is an enormously complex function. It involves the entire body in some fairly intense physical, mental, and emotional activity before, during, and after the act itself. The kind of sexual performance that we all dream about is a high-level function. It is possible only when the organs and glands are in good working order.

This is not to say that you must be in world-class or Olympic shape in order to have a terrific sex life. On the contrary, there's evidence that excessive training will weaken you sexually, not strengthen you. (More about this later.)

HIGH-DENSITY NUTRITION CAN MAKE A DIFFERENCE

The approach of most nutritionists writing about sex is that everything that supports good health will support good sex. That's true, but it doesn't satisfy our need to know more about what we can do for our sex life. In this chapter we are going to take the approach that because good sex is a high-level function, it is possible and sometimes necessary to lend some extra nutritional support to the organs and glands that play important roles in sex.

Those organs are:

- The brain and nervous system. We've all heard that the major sex organ is the brain. It's true. Desire and potency begin in the brain and the nervous system—and without the nervous system, they wouldn't lead to very much. The nervous system is actually the focal point of sex. If those nerve impulses aren't in touch with what's going on, nothing's going to go on.
- The adrenals and other endocrine glands. The adrenal glands are probaby next in importance, after the brain, to good sex. The adrenals control any excited state the body gets itself into in response to stimulation. That stimulation can be the proverbial angry boss or an amorous member of the opposite sex, and the response can be "make war, make tracks, or make love." In any case, the adrenals secrete hormones, including sex hormones, that make each activity possible by orchestrating the heart, nerves, muscles, and sex organs to do the

right jobs at the right times. If the adrenals are weak, libido and potency are also diminished.

- The sex glands. The ovaries and the testes are, of course, also vital to sex. These glands secrete hormones that control sexual desire, potency, and fertility.
- The prostate gland is probably the organ that slows down or causes trouble in more men's sex lives than any other organ. But it may also be the organ that, properly supported, may be the key to higher potency.
- The sex organs themselves. The mucous membranes of the vagina are vital to an enjoyable sex life, not only because they provide lubrication, but also because they help protect against infection.

SUPPORT YOUR SEX ORGANS WITH GOOD NUTRITION

For many women, the ability of their mucous membranes to keep vaginal tissues moist and strong is a limiting factor in how much and how often they can enjoy sex. The mucous membranes can become dried out and irritated, making sex painful and rendering the vagina more prone to infections. Vitamin A is the principal nutrient responsible for the health of the mucous membranes. Supplements of vitamin A stimulate the production of mucus and keep the membranes well lubricated and strong. Vitamin C, vitamin E, bioflavonoids, and zinc are also important to maintaining the mucous membranes.

Essential fatty acids, from evening primrose oil and fish oils will also help maintain the strength and proper lubrication of the sex organs. Adrenal hormones and sex hormones are made from essential fatty acids, so adequate dietary levels are required for a good sex life.

Beta-carotene, folic acid, vitamin E, and selenium are important nutrients for protecting the interior female sex organs, especially the cervix, from abnormal cell growths leading to cancer. Carotene can not only prevent cervical dysplasia (abnormal cell growth), but it can actually help reverse it.

Vitamin E supplements can help relieve breast cysts, which are believed to increase a women's risk of breast cancer. Drinking coffee increases the risk of these lumps developing in the breasts. Many women can get rid of these lumps just by eliminating coffee and other sources of caffeine from their diet.

SUPER SUPPLEMENTS FOR YOUR SEX GLANDS

The sex glands secrete hormones that stimulate the sex drive and potency. Nutritional support of the sex glands should include B vitamins for their normalizing effects on hormones, zinc for its supportive and stimulatory powers (more about this shortly), and the amino acids, glycine, alanine, and glutamic acid. The amino acid arginine, in doses ranging from 3 to 10 grams per day, has been shown to increase sperm count and motility.

THE RETURN OF THE SEX VITAMIN

What about vitamin E, the sex vitamin? Vitamin E is called the sex vitamin because it *is* vital to reproduction. Vitamin E is required for production of hormones and hormonelike prostaglandins that stimulate sexual activity. Without adequate vitamin E, spontaneous abortions occur in both animals and humans, and the vitamin has been used to prevent miscarriages. Vitamin E can also improve circulation, which is certainly a factor in sex.

But is there actually any evidence that vitamin E can

enhance sex in more, let us say, tangible ways? Can vitamin E earn its reputation as the sex vitamin?

Thanks to recent research, the answer is Yes—at least for women. Here's how:

When vitamin E levels are raised, the levels of female sex hormone, estrogen, also rise. So do the adrenal sex hormones. As these hormone levels go up, the female sex response may be heightened right along with them. Recent studies have shown that boosting these hormone levels results in an increase in the frequency of sexual intercourse and higher self-rated sexual gratification scores. In other words, vitamin E can mean more and better sex. The sex vitamin has returned.

THE SECRET BEHIND A TIME-HONORED APHRODISIAC

Vitamin E may indeed be a nutritional aphrodisiac. But when a man and woman begin the evening by sitting down to a romantic candlelit dinner, no one wants to gaze longingly into the other's eyes and whisper, "I'll have the vitamin E."

Now both of the authors of this book have certainly been known to pull out a little plastic bag of supplements at the end of a restaurant meal and begin swallowing tablets and capsules, while others at the table shake their heads and mutter that "they certainly do believe in it!"

But not when we're trying to set a romantic mood.

At those times, we want to surrender to romantic tradition and order a real food that will suggest, and maybe even help create, an amorous mood. If the menu allows, we'll order mussels, or oysters, whose reputation as an aphrodisiac goes back thousands of years.

For good reason. It seems that romantic tradition is converging with science, because mussels and oysters may actually fulfill their role as an aphrodisiac. Mussels are very high in mucopolysaccharides, which are natural substances that, together with collagen, form the glue that holds together all body tissues. Mucopolysaccharides support the strength and elasticity of the tissues and membranes, regulate the transfer of nutrients, help control inflammation, and protect against infection.

And, one more thing: They boost the male's production of seminal fluid, and thereby, increase sex drive and potency.

So it's no accident that mussels and oysters are legendary aphrodisiacs, because they contain extremely high concentrations of mucopolysaccharides. Some enterprising scientists made a list of all the legendary aphrodisiac foods and discovered that many of them were also very high in mucopolysaccharides.

Where does this leave our romantic diners? Well, we're going to assume that the lady has been taking her vitamin E regularly, as the gentleman has been faithfully taking his mucopolysaccharides. Our only problem then is one of etiquette: Who orders the mussels?

SUPPORT YOUR GLANDS DIRECTLY

Glandular supplements may also help enhance your sex life. In particular, ovarian substance is potentially supportive for women and testicular substance for both men and women, because testosterone stimulates the sex drive in both males and females. Because the sex drive is, in part, regulated by adrenal hormones, adrenal substance may also be useful. Vitamin A, vitamin C, and pantothenic acid are the principal supporters of the adrenal gland. Pantothenic acid and vitamin C both assist in the production of adrenal hormones.

For further support of endocrine function, pituitary and thyroid substance may help stimulate all the glands to function better, including the sex glands.

STIMULATE THE PRIMARY SEX ORGAN— THE BRAIN

The B vitamins, magnesium, potassium, and calcium support the function of the nervous system, including the balancing of moods, the excitability of the muscles and nerves, coordination, sensitivity, and mental and emotional energy.

Neurotransmitters in the brain control a wide range of activities, mental abilities, and moods. Certain nutritional substances can alter the balance of neurotransmitters, and thereby affect sex drive and potency. Choline improves memory and alertness, and so may enhance sexual function. The amino acid tryptophan produces a relaxed, antidepressed state that may be conducive to sex.

STIMULATE THE BRAIN'S OWN APHRODISIAC

Phenylalanine and tyrosine also support a brain environment that may encourage good sex. Phenylalanine increases brain levels of a chemical called phenyethylamine, or PEA. PEA is believed to be the body's own aphrodisiac; the body makes it directly from phenylalanine. PEA is known to be low in people who are depressed and who have low sex drives.

ZINC, THE SEX MINERAL

Last—and for a man, at least, perhaps foremost—comes zinc . . . and the prostate gland.

The prostate is responsible for secreting prostatic fluid,

which is a major component of the male ejaculate. Because of its key anatomical position, wrapped around the urethra, nothing can clamp down on a rollicking sex life faster than a swollen prostate. To make matters worse, the prostate can become swollen for many reasons. One of those reasons is infection. Another is lack of use. And another is . . . a rollicking sex life. The prostate appears to become swollen if it's used too much (or, at least, more than it's accustomed to being used) and if it's not used enough. Apparently the gland thrives on regularity.

But, fortunately, it thrives on one other thing: zinc. The wonder mineral zinc may be the closest thing to a nutritional aphrodisiac. The highest concentration of zinc in the male body is in the prostate and the prostatic fluid. With every ejaculation, a man loses some of that zinc. As the body manufactures more prostatic fluid, it requires more zinc.

We know that zinc is a very important mineral for the prostate gland. Zinc supplements can help prevent and relieve a condition know as benign prostatic hypertrophy, which is a fancy way of saying "a swollen or inflamed prostate gland."

But we believe zinc does even more.

ZINC MAY DIRECTLY STIMULATE THE SEX DRIVE

It's known that zinc is necessary for sexual maturation in both males and females. The sex glands require zinc for growth and normal operation. Zinc is required for the manufacture of sex hormones. Zinc-deficient children suffer growth and sexual retardation, but when zinc is restored to their diets, they grow by leaps and bounds. There have been some startling cases of growth- and sexually retarded young people catching up and gaining full sexual maturity in a matter of weeks after receiving zinc supplements.

We know that zinc deficiency can also hamper sexual

potency in an adult male. Zinc supplements have been used successfully to restore testosterone levels and sexual potency in men who have zinc deficiencies owing to renal dialysis. Zinc supplements can also increase testosterone levels and sperm count.

We believe that zinc not only stimulates testosterone and increases sperm count, but that it also stimulates the prostate gland. The combined effect is not only to increase sex drive but also to improve potency. Zinc's effect on male libido and potency is one that has not been tested—and probably cannot be tested—scientifically, through double-blind trials. But we've heard the reports of people who have experienced the effects of zinc supplementation on their sex lives. And we've experienced the sex-enhancing effects of zinc ourselves.

One word of caution: Zinc is a trace mineral and is effective in small doses. Zinc supplements of 25 to 100 mg. should be sufficient to restore adequate zinc levels, unless you have a specific problem with zinc metabolism or absorption. Higher doses may actually suppress immunity, decrease the body's copper stores, and raise cholesterol levels. Many people make the mistake of taking their zinc supplements with meals high in fiber, especially whole grains. Because the fiber in many whole grains interferes with zinc absorption, it's best to take zinc supplements at relatively low-fiber meals.

WILL ZINC STIMULATE WOMEN, TOO?

Will zinc supplements stimulate female libido and potency, as well? Insofar as zinc stimulates testosterone function in females, the answer is yes. But does it stimulate an equivalent of a prostate gland? Perhaps it does. But because anatomy books do not acknowledge the existence of a female prostate gland, no researcher is going to study whether zinc (or anything else) stimulates it. (Unfortunately, modern medicine has not explored the physiology of female sexuality as much as it has male sexuality. Witness the ongoing controversy over whether or not women have a "G-spot," or whether they do, in fact, ejaculate.)

In any case, zinc has enough benefits for both male and female to warrant it being an important part of any supplement program.

EXERCISE—DON'T OVERDO IT

Every book or magazine article about sexual function is obligated to say that exercise is the best thing for your sex life. It is—and it isn't. Exercise does reduce stress, strengthen the entire body, and improve functioning of all systems, including sexual functioning.

But only up to a point. Exercise at or above training levels can actually diminish hormone levels and reduce sexual drive and potency. Your muscles, lungs, and heart may be in world class shape, but perhaps you just don't have the hormones! Many women, for example, have found that they can turn off their periods merely by running a certain number of miles per week.

A natural reason for this phenomenon can be found in evolution. For most of the time we humans have been on earth, we've been a very mobile race. We've been stationary in cities and towns for less than 1 percent of our total evolutionary existence. When we were nomadic hunter-gatherers, there must have been entire seasons when we had to migrate in order to find food. Pregnancy and infant care would have been a distinct disadvantage during these long migrations. And the often near-starvation of the migration would certainly not have been the best condition in which to carry a child. So the body evolved in such a way that sustained, regular physical activity diminished levels of sex hormones and reduced not only sex drive, but fertility as well.

The tip here is to exercise for fitness, but if you're interested in stimulating your sex life, don't overdo it.

The case of Polly, a thirty-four-year-old marketing manager for a Silicon Valley computer manufacturer, provides an example of how Beyond Vitamins supplements can improve a sex life. Polly came to me with a problem that has become the bane of sexually active people in the 1970s and 1980s: genital herpes. Every six to eight weeks, this tall, attractive woman with long ash-blond hair broke out with painful herpes sores in her genital area and buttocks.

I explained to Polly that there was, as yet, no cure for herpes, but that there were some nutritional measures she could take that might reduce the frequency and the severity of the attacks.

Polly, an educated professional woman, knew enough about nutrition to stay away from junk food—except for her one indulgence, which was chocolate. She confessed that she even had T-shirts and pillows that announced that she was a "chocolate freak." Aside from that, Polly's diet was mostly natural foods. She loved salads with nuts and seeds added for the extra crunch.

Before I put Polly on a supplement program, I told her there were a few items in her diet that would have to go. Polly was right in suspecting the chocolate as the first culprit. Not only was the sugar weakening her immune system, but it also hampered the action of lysine, a natural antiherpes amino acid that I planned to prescribe for her. Along with the chocolate would have to go the nuts and seeds as well. Nuts, seeds, and chocolate contain too much arginine, an amino acid that, in and of itself, is actually good for the immune system. But it also competes with lysine, so for someone who's trying to maximize the effectiveness of the lysine they're taking, nuts, seeds, and chocolate are out.

Polly was advised to take the full spectrum of basic multivitamin-minerals, plus the immune-boosting supplements in Chapter 5 (with the exception of arginine). Also, Polly took 1,500 to 2,000 mg. of lysine every morning before breakfast.

Polly reported almost immediate improvement. The pain in her current outbreak was much relieved, and healing took place faster. Three months later, she reported that she had suffered only one outbreak. After two years, Polly says she has suffered only three outbreaks, and these during times of extreme stress. But, even so, they were not as serious as her previous attacks.

The Beyond Vitamins Multisupplement
for a Better Sex Life

For additional information on how to design your personal Beyond Vitamins Program, see Chapter 15.

VITAMINS
Vitamin A	10,000 I.U.
Carotene	25,000 I.U.
Thiamine	50 mg.
Riboflavin	50 mg.
Niacin	50 mg.
Pyridoxine	50 mg.
Pantothenic Acid	100–300 mg.
Folate	400 mcg.
B_{12}	100 mcg.
Biotin	400 mcg.
Choline	250 mg.
Inositol	100–200 mg.
PABA	100 mg.
Vitamin C	1,000–3,000 mg.
Bioflavonoids	200–1,000 mg.
Vitamin E	200–600 I.U.

MINERALS
Calcium	500 mg.
Magnesium	400 mg.
Potassium	100 mg.
Selenium	100–200 mcg.
Zinc	15–100 mg.

AMINO ACIDS
Alanine	100–250 mg.
Glutamic Acid	100–250 mg.
Glycine	100–250 mg.

Tyrosine	100–500 mg.
Tryptophan	500–1,500 mg.
	(taken separately)
Phenylalanine	500–1,500 mg.
	(taken separately)

GLANDULARS

Adrenal	50 mg.
Testicular	50 mg
Ovarian	50 mg.
Thyroid	50 mg.
Pituitary	50 mg.

OTHERS

GLA	40 mg.
EPA (fish oil)	500 mg.
Mucopolysaccharides	100–200 mg.

CHAPTER
10 Relieve Your
Allergies

A DECADE AGO, to most people the word *allergy* meant hay fever, or respiratory distress caused by particles of dust, pollen, or hair floating in the air. Few people were aware that the concept of allergy was being extended to the very foods we eat.

Allergic reactions are caused by the immune system, which has two major responsibilities. The first is to scrutinize organisms, substances, and particles that invade the body through the respiratory system, the circulatory system, the mucous membranes, or the digestive tract. Once scrutinized, the immune system is supposed to identify the invader as either part of the body or not part of the body: self or not self. Once an invader is identified as not self, the immune system's second task is to declare war on the invader. The immune system doesn't wait to see whether the invader's intentions are harmless. Once it's identified as not self, the immune system attacks it.

Being allergic to something means your immune system has become sensitized so that it identifies that substance or thing as not self and, in effect, declares war on it every time you come in contact with it. The immune system has a very efficient memory so that it never forgets an invader with whom it's done battle. This is a remarkable ability, one that saves our lives many times over.

But in many people this immune memory also causes allergies. The immune system is primed by genetic factors or sensitized early in life to recognize a normally harmless substance such as pollen or fur as a danger, and reacts with an immune show of force that can leave you feeling miserable.

THE AGING IMMUNE SYSTEM'S MEMORY SLIPS

There's also evidence that as we get older the immune system's memory starts to slip, and it starts forgetting faces, so to speak. Over a long period, a little at a time, it mistakes self for not self and attacks our own body.

All allergies are a form of heightened sensitivity. Normally, the body should not react to certain substances in such a way as to cause the profound discomfort brought on by allergies. Try telling this to someone in the throes of a hay fever attack.

Although many physicians resisted the evidence for a long time, we now know that people can also become allergic to common, everyday foods. In fact, the more common the food is, the more likely it is to cause allergic reactions. We'll explain.

FOOD ALLERGIES—WHY?

The reasons for food allergies are slightly different than the reasons behind inhalant and contact allergies. We know that the body has no positive use for inhaled pollens, cat dander, or paint and diesel fumes. But why should the immune system attack your corn flakes?

The reason is that corn flakes, or the milk you consumed with them—or both—do not belong in your bloodstream in quite the form that your digestive system is allowing them to enter. Normally, these foods would be broken down sufficiently so that when the nutrients were absorbed into your blood, the proteins would be small enough to be easily utilized. Now, however, those proteins are getting into your blood in larger-than-normal form. Once there, they provoke an attack by the immune system, the kind of attack that leaves a memory behind forever. So, if corn is the offending food, every time you eat corn flakes, corn chips, or anything that has even trace amounts of proteins recognizable as coming from corn—including corn syrup—your immune system may go on the march.

STEP ONE: INCOMPLETE DIGESTION

How do those larger-than-normal protein molecules get through? Two ways. First, the digestive system does not complete its job of breaking them down. The main reason for that is an insufficiency of digestive enzymes and/or hydrochloric acid. Perhaps your digestive glands are not producing enough enzymes. Or maybe you simply didn't chew your food enough, so there were too many large pieces that were impossible to break down completely.

If we don't have enough digestive enzymes, food particles will not be broken down small enough for adequate absorption of nutrients to take place. Some of the nutrients from our food and from our supplements can be wasted.

This becomes a serious problem as we get older. After the age of 40, levels of hydrochloric acid and digestive enzymes begin to decrease. So as we get older, we're more likely to become victims of poor absorption and multiple nutritional deficiencies—even though we may be eating a diet that was adequate for us when we were younger.

As we continue to be undernourished, the situation worsens because the body's ability to produce adequate amounts of enzymes is further weakened.

That's easy enough to understand. But how do we explain the seemingly contradictory statement that inadequate digestion promotes the absorption of unfriendly molecules? The answer is simple. Inadequate digestion allows many undigested, larger-than-normal protein molecules to be passed along to the intestines. Most of these larger molecules become waste, but not all of them.

Many of them wind up in the bloodstream.

STEP TWO: THE LEAKY GUT

Once those troublesome, larger-than-normal protein molecules get past the places where enzymes are supposed to break them down, how do they get into the bloodstream? Well, it appears they go right through the walls of the intestine. We once thought that these walls were a perfect barrier, or filter, allowing only small, easily utilized proteins through into the blood. We now know otherwise. The gut may be a leaky barrier, allowing large proteins to sneak through all the time—especially when that intestinal wall has been weakened by marginal nutrition or inflammation. (We know, for example, that low levels of vitamin A and zinc can make the leaky gut even worse.)

STEP THREE: THE IMMUNE SYSTEM DECLARES WAR

And once those proteins get into the blood, the trouble really starts; the immune system attacks them. This immune reaction can produce a wide range of symptoms. Maybe you'll feel tired, or vaguely ill. You may get a headache, become depressed, experience mood swings or digestive upsets. Your skin may break out. Because your absorption of nutrients is further inhibited, you may suffer deficiency symptoms.

THE BIRTH OF A CRAVING

But that's not all that happens. The adrenals and other glands are also stimulated, and the brain and its balance of neurotransmitters can also be affected. The mood-altering effects of incomplete breakdown products entering the bloodstream can cause a mild, temporary elation, a burst of energy, or a general analgesia or numbing of pain. In some people, the stimulation is so great that an impossible-to-ignore stress or "fight or flight" reaction occurs. Their heart flutters or pounds, their blood pressure goes up, their breathing increases, their muscles tense.

In some people, the stimulation results in a barely perceptible "high" when the body secretes other adrenal hormones to modulate the initial reaction. Many people become addicted to this "high," which is usually followed by a "low," or withdrawal symptoms, including depression, nervousness, irritability, fatigue, and compulsive behavior.

WHY WE CRAVE CERTAIN FOODS

This explains why we're often addicted to foods that give us an allergic reaction or, in other words, why our favorite foods are the foods to which we're allergic. Any food we are drawn to compulsively is one that's likely to soothe or stimulate us by provoking a hormonal response—as the allergic reaction does.

An unfortunate few are so caught up in this compulsive cycle that they experience the withdrawal symptoms without noticing that the corn chips they ate made them feel good, before they plunged them into any of a wide range of symptoms, including mild confusion, rage, headaches, fatigue, dizziness, irritability, hyperactivity, depression, mood swings, muddled thinking, and psychotic symptoms.

Adrenal glands that have become exhausted from constantly dealing with allergic responses produce fatigue, loss of sex drive, and susceptibility to infections. Other affected organs might produce blood sugar swings, high blood pressure, vague pains, and so on.

The only way to break the cycle of craving-stimulation is to prevent incomplete breakdown products from entering the bloodstream. There are three ways to do this, and all three methods are usually combined for the best therapeutic effect. First, all offending and potentially offending foods are temporarily withdrawn from the diet. Second, digestion is made more efficient through the use of digestive enzymes. Finally, through the use of nutritional supplements, the "leaky gut" is encouraged to heal and become a more effective barrier.

AND BEHIND THE SCENES— INFLAMMATION

Food allergies not only cause inflammation, but they also thrive on it. Invariably affected are the digestive organs themselves. Inflamed intestines make it that much easier for large food proteins to pass through, thus aggravating the problem. Finally, a distracted immune system spends its vital energy fighting off imagined threats and so grows less efficient at protecting us from genuine dangers.

TEST YOURSELF TO FIND OUT

How do you know if you have a food allergy?

If you regularly feel tired, get a headache, or have mental symptoms such as depression, confusion, difficulty concentrating within a few hours after eating, there's a good chance that you're allergic to one or more foods in that meal. If you experience a lot of gas or bloating, it's a sign that incompletely digested food is reaching the bacteria in your intestines, making food allergies more likely to occur. If you sometimes feel better, more clearheaded and energetic, after you skip a meal, it's a good sign of food allergies. By not eating, you've allowed the allergic reaction to allergenic foods to "clear."

Finally, food allergies can also cause symptoms identical to inhalant allergies—sniffles, sinus drainage, sore throat, and stuffy head. If you experience persistent symptoms such as this, and there are no environmental causes, you may have food allergies.

There are several laboratory tests designed to diagnose food allergies. But by far the best method—and the most accurate—is the test you perform on yourself by removing all suspected foods from your diet for four days, then reintroducing them one at a time, one every day or two, while keeping track of your symptoms. You may have to go on a modified diet for a few days, eating only hypoallergenic foods such as fresh vegetables, rice, and pure water in order to detoxify or "clear" the reaction-producing hormones and toxic by-products of the allergic reaction from your body.

THE BEYOND VITAMINS APPROACH TO ALLERGIES

Treatment of food allergies varies. Some physicians and nutritionists believe that it's necessary that you permanently avoid your allergenic foods. We believe this is often too extreme, although you will need to avoid them for some period of time. In about 10 percent of cases, where reactions are potentially dangerous, permanent avoidance is recommended. But for the remainder, which are not permanent allergies, a treatment program enforcing permanent avoidance ignores the potential benefits you might gain from a supplement program designed to help you deal with your allergies. Our Beyond Vitamins approach to allergies can help you:

- Increase your digestive efficiency to prevent the passing of large protein molecules into the intestines
- Reduce your inflammatory response in the gut and elsewhere in order to reduce your allergic reaction not only to foods but also to pollens, dust, molds, and other environmental allergens
- Repair your leaky gut to minimize the amount of undigested protein entering the bloodstream
- Increase the efficiency of your immune system, to prevent its weakening by your allergies
- Strengthen your adrenal glands to prevent the cycle of allergy withdrawal from exhausting you
- Increasing the efficiency of your body's detoxifying ability, to lessen the impact of the allergic response

Understand that these supplements are meant to augment, not substitute for, a comprehensive allergy-treatment plan designed by your doctor.

INCREASE YOUR DIGESTIVE EFFICIENCY

Fundamental to any prevention or relief of food allergies is your digestive efficiency. Digestive enzymes, especially pancreatin, will help break down food particles. And betaine hydrochloride is a good digestive aid to increase the hydrochloric acid in your stomach.

If you're not digesting your food completely, you probably do not have enough pancreatic enzymes. The pancreas secretes protein-, starch-, and fat-digesting enzymes into the small intestine in response to the acidity of the stomach contents. So if your stomach is deficient in hydrochloric acid, the food entering the intestines will not be sufficiently acidic, and your pancreas will not secrete enough enzymes to digest the food properly.

Many factors can interfere with proper, complete digestion. If you're under stress or upset in any way before or during a meal, hydrochloric or enzyme secretion may be diminished. If a meal does not contain enough amino acids, especially tryptophan and/or phenylalanine, enzyme secretion may be lowered. Illness or chronic malnutrition will also decrease your ability to produce enzymes. The pancreas adapts to your habitual diet, but if you switch diets quickly, before the gland can adapt its patterns of enzyme secretion, incomplete digestion can result. Finally, as we get older, our ability to manufacture hydrochloric acid and digestive enzymes decreases significantly.

NUTRIENTS TO HEAL AND SUPPORT YOUR DIGESTIVE ORGANS

The following glandular supplements may help heal and maintain your digestive organs: pancreas substance, duodenum substance, and stomach substance.

Vitamin A, vitamin C, zinc, and the B vitamins, especially niacin, are also required to maintain the integrity of the digestive system.

A CRUCIAL SUPPLEMENT THAT'S FREE

One more supplement that doesn't come in a bottle: chewing. Add about 50 percent more chewing before you swallow your food. We learned in grammar school that digestion begins in the mouth. But many of us forget and fail to take full advantage of our own digestive standard equipment. The advantage of extra chewing is that it breaks

up food particles and gives your enzymes more surface area
to work on, thus increasing the efficiency of digestion.

NUTRIENTS TO REDUCE INFLAMMATION

By reducing inflammation we hope to de-escalate the immune system's attack on the allergenic substance, whether
it's a food or cat dander.

Vitamin C and the bioflavonoids are natural and very
effective anti-inflammatory agents. Bioflavonoids can actually prevent the mast cells from discharging histamine
and other inflammatory substances. Combined with pineapple enzyme bromelain and other enzymes trypsin and
chymotrypsin, you have an anti-inflammatory supplement
that may be more effective than aspirin and other nonsteroidal drugs—without the side effects or drug hazards.

The bioflavonoids, vitamin C, vitamin A, and zinc will
also help heal and strengthen the walls of the intestine to
prevent the leaky gut that allows large protein molecules
into the blood. And their enzyme-deactivating, anti-inflammatory effects will help decrease the inflammation pro-
voked by allergens that do get through.

The B vitamins, especially pantothenic acid and B_6, can
also be effective anti-inflammatory supplements, through
their support of the adrenal glands.

Edible oils from fish oils and essential fatty acids (evening primrose oil) are also effective anti-inflammatories.
Both of these oils promote the release of anti-inflammatory
prostaglandins of the PG1 and PG3 series.

The amino acid tyrosine is beneficial in reducing the intensity and frequency of hay fever attacks.

Glandular supplements, spleen substance, and adrenal
substance may also help reduce the inflammation of allergic reactions.

CONTROL YOUR
ALLERGY-FEEDBACK SYSTEM

The amino acid histidine may also be helpful in reducing the allergic reaction in hay fever and other inhalant allergies. We know of people who have tried it and reported that their hay fever disappeared. In one case it took only one week.

If it works, it does so by a seeming paradox. Histidine is a precursor of histamine. That's right, histamine is the chemical that the mast cells release in an allergic reaction —it's the chemical that causes all the trouble. So why does taking a supplement that forms histamine relieve allergies? It should make allergies worse!

The body has a feedback mechanism for histamine. If it senses that it's producing too much, it will stimulate suppressor cells that shut down histamine release. Theoretically, the histidine supplement tricks the feedback mechanism into shutting off the histamine.

We add a few words of caution here. Try histidine only under a physician's careful monitoring. It may backfire on some people and produce more histamine and, hence, more violent allergic reactions. Also, histidine tends to pull zinc out of the body. If you take histidine, make sure your zinc levels are adequate.

NUTRIENTS TO REPAIR THE LEAKY GUT

The cells of the bowel wall are replenished every three days, so there is a very rapid turnover of cells. It is as if you have a constant healing process going on, and the demand for nutrients is very high. Nutrients that can help you strengthen the integrity of your bowel wall include: vitamin A, which replenishes the protective layer of mucus and mucous membranes of the bowel wall. Vitamin C and zinc are also principal nutrients for healing. Bioflavonoids and mucopolysaccharides help maintain the strength of all membranes. Protein and nucleic acids are also of value for healing and in any situation involving rapid turnover of cells.

Glandular supplements of duodenum and stomach substance may also be valuable in regenerating the intestinal barrier.

INCREASE THE EFFICIENCY OF YOUR IMMUNE SYSTEM

Follow the instructions in our chapter on boosting your immune system (Chapter 5). You might think it contradictory to boost your immune system when it's your immune system that's causing all the trouble. It's not contradictory, however, for two reasons. Making your immune system more efficient means that you may not only make it stronger, but also better at deciding what is actually a threat to your body. As we get older, this ability drops off somewhat—even to the point where the immune system starts attacking the very body it's supposed to protect! When that happens, allergies get worse, not better. The supplements we recommend for boosting the immune system will also help it resist this tendency.

Second reason: Food allergies weaken the immune system. The immune system has enough to do fighting off an almost constant barrage of bacteria, viruses, and environmental junk that finds its way into our bodies without having to send troops into battle against breakfast, lunch, and dinner, too.

STRENGTHEN
YOUR ADRENAL GLANDS

Weak adrenal glands make allergies worse. Here's how: When the adrenals are strong and an allergen enters the body, the glands are able to secrete hormones that modulate the inflammatory response and reduce the discomfort. With many food allergies, for example, strong adrenal glands may render the allergic reaction imperceptible and, for practical purposes, of negligible importance.

When the glands are weak, however, they are unable to secrete enough of the hormones that modulate the reaction. As a result, the reaction has a greater, more unpleasant, and noticeable effect—and it may last longer. When the reaction is mild and short-lived, the chances for addiction or cravings developing are small. When the reaction is strong and lasts for a long time, the potential for addiction or cravings is high. We are compelled to hit the adrenals harder and harder in order to beat some modulating hormones out of them to reduce our symptoms.

To strengthen the adrenals, vitamins A, C, and pantothenic acid are the first team. Adrenal substance glandular supplements may also help heal and strengthen the adrenals.

NUTRIENTS TO INCREASE YOUR BODY'S
DETOXIFYING ABILITY

Allergic reactions flood the body with toxic chemicals and free radicals. The body's ability to withstand the direct assault of the allergic reaction, plus its ability to bounce back after the reaction, is largely determined by its ability to detoxify those noxious by-products.

The principal detoxifying organ of the body is the liver.

It's our nominee for Unsung Hero of the Body, for it not only detoxifies all kinds of gunk that passes through the body—some of which is produced by the body, some of which is not—but it also stores energy, converts protein into carbohydrates, and manufactures many chemicals the body can't live without.

To give credit where credit is due, and also to give a supplement its due, the first supplement for the liver is . . . liver. It's no accident that liver was among the very first supplements, if not the first. Among the initial modern scientific nutritional experiments were experiments demonstrating that liver contained substances that had a beneficial effect on health and fitness, substances that were not among the vitamins or minerals, substances that we have yet to identify.

The beneficial nutrients that we know are in liver include: vitamin A, the B vitamins, vitamin D, all the minerals, all the essential amino acids, nucleic acids, and liver substance itself.

Other supplements to boost your detoxifying ability include the following:

The antioxidants carotene, vitamin C, vitamin E, zinc, DMG (dimethylglycine), and the amino acids cysteine and methionine will aid detoxification in the liver and elsewhere in the body. Toxic chemicals often do their damage by promoting free radical oxidative damage. These antioxidants neutralize the free radicals.

Two more "supplements" that will aid detoxification are a high-starch diet and water. There are two things the liver needs more of than anything else to carry out detoxification: water and glycogen, the stored form of blood sugar. The liver needs glycogen in order to form glucuronic acid, one of the major detoxifying chemicals. So a liver that's full of glucose detoxifies better. A diet that contains large amounts of complex carbohydrates will fill the liver with glycogen.

Because the by-products of detoxification are literally washed out of the body through the liver, kidneys, and skin, we need to drink plenty of water. It's true, a lot of these antioxidants are going to be washed out right along with the toxins, and that is the way you want it. Nothing is wasted, because they keep on neutralizing those free radicals all along the way. Remember, we're not entirely safe from these chemicals until they're in the toilet. Think of your "excess" nutrients as a kind of "police escort" that keeps these chemicals out of trouble on the way out.

Here is a case in which Beyond Vitamins supplements were useful in reducing allergies.

Clara was a thirty-six-year-old woman who had moved to Marin County, a suburb of San Francisco, about two years earlier. During her first year here, Clara started to suffer from allergies. Her symptoms were mild: only some sniffles during April and May.

Why did Clara's allergies wait until she was 36 years old before coming out? Well, first of all, Clara had definitely come from an allergic family. By Clara's recollection, her mother "always carried a handkerchief and was blowing her nose." Also, her younger sister had asthma.

But Clara had managed to escape allergies by living in a big city, where she was not exposed to trees and grass. All of that changed, of course, when she moved to Marin County, which is known for its lush forests and abundant greenery.

The second year, her symptoms grew much worse. Her nose ran all the time, her eyes were red, and she had sneezing fits in the morning. Worst of all, Clara had recurring fatigue and frequent headaches that seriously hampered her ability to function. She began to prefer staying indoors, where she felt somewhat better. She tried some over-the-counter medications, with only partial relief. She abandoned these drugs because they worsened her fatigue and made her mouth and eyes dry.

Clara's treatment was fairly straightforward. In addition to a basic supplement program, I (RM) gave her 1,000 to 4,000 mg. of vitamin C per day. During acute allergy attacks, I raised the dose to 6,000 to 10,000 mg. A person suffering from allergies benefits from vitamin C because it is an adrenal gland stimulant and natural antihistamine. High doses may cause gas, bloating, and diarrhea, but these may only be indications that the body has absorbed all that it needs. I instructed Clara to reduce her dose when these symptoms occurred. She reported that during acute attacks, the high doses of vitamin C seldom caused any side effects. That was an indication that she was absorbing all of the vitamin C.

Clara also took pantothenic acid, 200 to 500 mg. per day. During acute attacks she took up to 2,000 mg. Pantothenic acid also stimulates the adrenal glands to produce more allergy-modulating hormones. That much pantothenic acid can stimulate the bowel and produce gas and diarrhea, but is otherwise harmless. Clara also took niacin—200 to 500 mg. per day. Niacin can often inhibit allergic reactions by depleting the mast cells of histamine.

Clara also took some adrenal substance glandular supplements, which may also stimulate the adrenal glands. She reported that these helped. She was not made totally allergy-free, but she improved to the point where she could carry on a normal life and enjoy her home.

Beyond Vitamins Multisupplement for Allergies

For additional information on how to design your personal Beyond Vitamins Program, see Chapter 15.

VITAMINS

Vitamin A	10,000–20,000 I.U.
Carotene	25,000 I.U.
Thiamine	50 mg.
Riboflavin	50 mg.
Niacin	50–500 mg.
Pyridoxine	50 mg.
Pantothenic acid	100–500 mg.
Folate	400 mcg.

VITAMINS

B₁₂	100 mcg.
Biotin	400 mcg.
Choline	250 mg.
Inositol	100 mg.
PABA	100 mg.
Vitamin C	2,000–8,000 mg.
Bioflavonoids	500–4,000 mg.
Vitamin E	200–400 I.U.

MINERALS

Zinc	30–75 mg.

AMINO ACIDS

Methionine	100 mg.
Cysteine	100 mg.
Glutathione	100 mg.
Tyrosine	500–1,000 mg.

GLANDULARS

Adrenal	50–500 mg.
Pancreas	50 mg.
Thymus	50 mg.
Stomach	50 mg.
Duodenum	50 mg.
Liver	500 mg.

ENZYMES

Betaine HCL	100 mg.
Pancreatin	100 mg.
Papain	100 mg.
Bromelain	100 mg.
Bile factors	100 mg.

OTHERS

EPA and/or DHA	500 mg.
GLA	40–240 mg.
Mucopolysaccharides	100–200 mg.
DMG	100 mg.

CHAPTER

11 New Keys To Unlock Better Health for Women

RIGHT NOW, calcium is in. The media are singing the praises of calcium as if it had just been discovered yesterday that women lose bone density at a faster rate than men, that this demineralization of bone is dangerous, and that calcium supplements can prevent it. Although it's true that the newsmagazines, the TV and radio networks, and a hefty proportion of the medical profession may have discovered these facts only recently, the basic research has been performed, published, and written about for the past 10 to 15 years.

There's no question as to the value of this increased publicity. Millions of women who might have gone on slowly losing the strength in their bones are now alerted to the problem and have the information to do something about it.

ARE THERE OTHER VITAL NUTRIENTS WOMEN NEED?

But it has to make you wonder: Are there other supplements women should be taking to help prevent serious problems? Is there information about women's nutrition that is not secret or fringe or doubtful, but is solid medical-nutritional news that simply has not reached the network news desks, the newspapers, or the newsmagazines?

The answer is yes. There is a lot of information about nutrition that might help many women live healthier, longer, more vigorous lives, if only they had access to it. Our plan in this chapter is to provide that access.

TODAY'S WOMAN HAS SPECIAL REQUIREMENTS

Women have special nutritional needs. Their special health problems require different supplements, for different reasons. Our intent in this chapter is not to separate women's needs from men's. On the contrary, the other chapters in this book apply to women at least as much as they apply to men.

Women are a very busy group of people! There are more than 90 million adult women in the United States, and more than half of them hold down full or part-time jobs outside the home. Of the 40 million or so who are not part of the "labor force," about 30 million are homemakers. More than half of all working women are married. Thirty million women have children under eighteen living at home—and 60 percent of working women belong to that group. Also, more than half of all women are on a diet, exercising regularly, drinking alcoholic beverages, and taking supplements. And whereas women have long enjoyed an advantage over men in longevity, increased cigarette smoking is helping women catch up with men and die just as young.

These statistics suggest that our chapters on maximum performance, dieting, sex, and basic stress supplements will be useful to most women.

Modern life seems to shortchange women when it comes to fulfilling their nutritional needs. Study after study turns up widespread deficiencies of vital nutrients among women.

TOO MANY WOMEN ARE POORLY NOURISHED

Nutritional surveys involving diet analysis and blood and tissue tests for nutrient status have found the following deficiencies in women:

- B_6 and iron-deficient diets in 90 percent of college women
- B-vitamin iron-, calcium-, magnesium-, and zinc-deficient diets in young women
- B_6-deficient diets in adolescent women, producing biochemical evidence of deficiencies
- Pantothenic acid deficiencies in pregnant women
- Diets deficient in zinc and copper
- Adult women selecting iron-deficient diets
- Diets that failed to supply enough calcium and magnesium to maintain body stores—the women were excreting more of these vital minerals than they were taking in
- Diets that failed to supply 70 percent of the RDA for zinc and folic acid were found in 70 percent of adult women; calcium and iron, 30 percent; and magnesium and B_6, 40 percent
- Other surveys by the USDA and others have found widespread deficiencies of calcium, iron, and magnesium, vitamin A, vitamin C, and B_6 among women.

WOMEN ARE SOMETIMES AT GREATER RISK

Some of these deficiencies are traceable to women's special needs. For example, pregnancy, childbirth, and lactation put women at risk for developing a wide range of nutritional deficiencies, including the B vitamins, iron, vitamin E, and vitamin C. Oral contraceptives use up more vitamins and minerals. Women also tend to eat less than men. The median caloric intake for women is 1,500 calories, which means that half of the women are eating more than 1,500 calories a day and half are eating less. Try designing a diet that supplies enough protein, vitamins, and minerals on only 1,500 calories a day—without the use of supplements!

For example, the median calcium intake for women is about 500 mg. per day. That means half of all women are getting less and half are getting more. Add to this statistic the fact that women do not absorb calcium as well as men and you will begin to understand how necessary supplements can be.

OSTEOPOROSIS—THE FULL STORY

As tacky as some of those advertisements and commercials for calcium supplements can be, they don't go far enough in detailing the full story of osteoporosis. The pictures show a stately young woman transformed before our eyes into a short, hunched-over old woman. What the ads don't tell us is that doctors once accepted this transformation as "just part of growing old," and told their women patients there was nothing that could be done. Often, the first symptom of osteoporosis that a physician would acknowledge was when the bones of a woman's leg, hip, or spine would simply shatter—spontaneously breaking under no more stress than standing up.

Osteoporosis kills. Fractures are a major cause of death in women over the age of fifty and, as the age increases, the number of deaths caused by fractures also increases. But these fractures, as well as the shortening of height caused by compression of the spine and the characteristic "dowager's hump" are not the first noticeable symptoms of osteoporosis—periodontal disease is. The jawbone is usually the first bone to lose minerals, and when the tooth-bearing bone is lost, the teeth are eventually loosened and finally lost.

Negative calcium balance, which means that the body is losing more calcium than it is taking in, causes not only the long, crippling disease of osteoporosis, but also some immediate problems. Low calcium balance is a factor in muscle cramps, fatigue, nervousness, irritability, high blood pressure and, we've recently learned, cancer.

CALCIUM IS NOT NEARLY ENOUGH

A complete program for the prevention or treatment of osteoporosis should involve more than calcium. The strength of the bones depends not only on calcium, but also on vitamin D, magnesium, vitamin C, zinc, and vitamin A. Physicians once believed that women started losing minerals from their bones solely because of decreasing levels of estrogen, the female hormone. We now know, however, that bone demineralization begins to occur before estrogen levels start to sink in middle age. In some women, osteoporosis begins as early as age 20.

Overall, estrogen may not be as much of a factor in bone demineralization as we once thought is was. Two other factors appear to be more important: calcium intake and the amount of exercise. Calcium supplements and exercise have each been shown to be at least as, and sometimes more, effective than estrogen supplements at maintaining and restoring bone density. Calcium supplements, with a small amount of vitamin D to aid in utilization of the calcium, not only can prevent osteoporosis, but also reverse the process and deposit minerals back into weakened bones.

One aspect of the osteoporosis story that's rarely reported is magnesium. Magnesium enhances calcium absorption and utilization while it decreases competition from phosphorus. Magnesium also ensures that calcium will be deposited in the bones and teeth rather than in the soft tissues of the body. No calcium supplementation should be without magnesium. Recent evidence suggests that manganese is also a key nutrient in maintaining strong bones.

USING YOUR BONES KEEPS THEM STRONG

Regular exercise is crucial to maintaining bone strength. Even the highly-fit astronauts were found to lose bone mass when they did not exercise for three days. It doesn't take much exercise, either. A one-hour walk, three or four times a week will serve to stimulate bone mineralization.

NO MORE MONTHLY MISERY

One thing many doctors seem to love to do more than just about anything else is to prescribe drugs to women. It has been reported that the single most common medical transaction is the administration of a mood-altering drug to a female patient by a male physician. When doctors discovered osteoporosis (but not calcium or exercise), they gave women estrogen. And when they discovered premenstrual syndrome, they once again prescribed hormones to "solve the problem."

Yet PMS can be alleviated without hormones or other drugs. A standard supplement program for PMS includes the following:

Evening primrose oil for essential fatty acids and fish oils for EPA and DHA. The fatty acids in EPO and fish oils stimulate the production of anti-inflammatory prostaglandins, which may help reduce or eliminate PMS symptoms.

Bioflavonoids and vitamin C are also effective anti-inflammatory supplements. Bioflavonoids, as reported in earlier chapters, can deactivate the enzymes that help produce inflammation. Bioflavonoids will also help reduce inflammation and excess menstrual bleeding by strengthening the walls of the small blood vessels.

There is some evidence that zinc is also anti-inflammatory. It strengthens the membranes and prevents "leaking" of body fluids through tissue barriers and blood vessels, a major cause of inflammation. In this case, zinc is also a valuable supplement for its ability to speed healing.

Calcium, magnesium, and potassium are also beneficial for their ability to balance the nerves, reduce irritability and fatigue resulting from tension, and relax the muscles. Cramps may also be relieved by magnesium.

The B vitamins, especially B_6, or pyridoxine, are especially important in PMS. The B vitamins help the body regulate hormones, and they support the brain and nervous system. Anytime there is tension, stress, loss of body fluids, or major metabolic shifts—as occur with PMS—there will also be increased need for B vitamins and other water-soluble nutrients, such as vitamin C. B_6 is used extensively to treat PMS. It has some effectiveness in preventing premenstrual tension and depression, but is used mostly to reduce swelling and water retention.

Any PMS supplement program should also include the antioxidants vitamin C, E, beta-carotene, and selenium for good measure. These nutrients help support the liver and aid in detoxifying noxious chemicals, even those produced by the body itself. Vitamin A is also a good idea, in that it is useful in relieving many menstrual problems, including heavy bleeding.

Amino acids may also be useful in PMS, especially when the symptoms arise from an imbalance of neurotransmitters in the brain. Female hormones are known to attach to receptors in the brain that normally serve to maintain neurotransmitter balance.

Tryptophan is an effective tranquilizer and is sometimes effective in relieving depression.

Phenylalanine is also a potent antidepressant. It can also be used to relieve cramps.

Anti-inflammatory enzymes bromelain and pancreatin are also helpful in relieving inflammatory PMS symptoms.

Iron supplements should also be taken to prevent anemia. Menstruating women are among the few groups that should regularly take iron supplements. (The other groups include pregnant and lactating women, and anyone who has suffered blood loss or injury.)

Glandular supplements: You might also try pituitary substance (or anterior pituitary substance). I (MR) have had cases of PMS that did not respond to the usual program but which did respond to anterior pituitary substance.

Diana was a typical example of a young career woman beset by PMS. Barely over 30, Diana was already vice president of a growing real estate investment firm. She managed 23 people in three departments and was responsible for over a billion dollars in capital. Yet she sat across from me in tears through most of our first meeting. The depression and anxiety that plagued her every month before her menstrual period were causing her to binge on junk food. Although she was able to manage her work, she was afraid that it was only a matter of time before her career was damaged. As it was, she took the two worst days off every month—and then came back to several days of "catch-up" work.

Diana was also taking birth control pills, which may have been making her problem worse by using up greater amounts of certain key nutrients, especially pyridoxine. The junk food Diana was binging on every month was also not helping, to put it mildly. By eating next to nothing for several days each month, Diana had been able to offset the fattening effects of her junk-food binging. But this pattern of "junk-food feast followed by famine" was obviously wreaking havoc with her nutritional state.

I advised Diana to begin with a basic multivitamin-mineral program and to try her best to stop her binging. To help with her depression and anxiety, I suggested she take either tyrosine or phenylalanine (500 mg. three times a day). This would also help her deal with her binging.

I also recommended a full PMS supplement program for her, which included all of the anti-PMS supplements in this chapter: B vitamins, vitamin C, bioflavonoids, vitamin E, calcium, magnesium, potassium, and evening primrose oil as a source of GLA.

Diana needed to do one more thing: exercise. She had grown up in southern California and had always driven to work. Although her apartment was within walking distance of the financial district, where her office was, she never walked to work. I recommended that she walk to work at least three times each week. I explained to her that exercise stimulates the body to produce its own antidepressants. Diana promised to try.

Two months later, Diana reported back that although she had experienced some difficulty in getting used to taking supplements, she did feel better. Her PMS symptoms had been greatly reduced in the previous month. Although she still felt depressed and anxious now and then, her mood swings were nowhere near as severe as before. She only occasionally felt compelled to binge on junk food, and most of the time she could control the urge. As for the walking, she said she had averaged twice a week. But she admitted that she did feel better on days when she walked.

Diana is now doing quite well. She reports that her PMS symptoms are gone—unless she slips up and doesn't take her supplements for a while. If she eats junk food, it's only when she is celebrating a very special event with friends. She says she walks to work every day, even on rainy days. And she has taken several vacations by using up the sick days that she doesn't need to spend on staying home with PMS.

DIET AND LIFESTYLE ARE IMPORTANT

Your diet and lifestyle can also affect your susceptibility to PMS. Food allergies, junk food, high-sugar or high-fat diet may all increase your risk of PMS. Many PMS sufferers find themselves drawn to certain foods, such as chocolate, when the time for their PMS symptoms approaches. These foods probably contribute to the problem. Sugar and fat, in particular, greatly disturb the body's mechanisms for maintaining balance in hormonal and metabolic systems. High body fat, for example, may raise estrogen levels. Proper amounts of protein are also required to maintain positive energy and moods. If your diet contains too much junk food and not enough protein, complex carbohydrates, fresh fruits, and vegetables, supplements may be of limited help.

MENOPAUSE RAISES CERTAIN REQUIREMENTS

All of the supplements recommended for PMS may also be useful for menopausal symptoms, with the following additional comments and recommendations:

With regard to taking calcium, vitamin D, and other supplements to prevent osteoporosis, if you are postmenopausal, it's still not too late to prevent further bone loss or, to some extent, reverse that which has taken place. Calcium and vitamin D supplements, with or without moderate exercise, have succeeded in reversing bone demineralization in people as old as eighty-nine years.

Bioflavonoids may help put out the fire of menopause, by virtue of their ability to deactivate inflammatory enzymes. Supplements of 1,200 mg per day of bioflavonoids, with an equal amount of vitamin C, can work better than estrogen supplements in relieving hot flashes in menopausal women. Vitamin E is also effective in relieving hot flashes.

Glandular supplements, particularly ovarian substance, may also be beneficial to menopausal women.

YOU DON'T HAVE TO BE MARRIED TO HAVE "HOUSEWIFE SYNDROME"

We are not responsible for the name of this affliction. The doctors who published the original report gave this name to a mixed bag of symptoms, including: morning tiredness, fatigue, lassitude, increasing exhaustion, vague pains, tension headaches, insomnia, and lower back pain—symptoms, which, by the way, they treated in men as well as women. The supplements that were successful in restoring energy and well-being in this syndrome were potassium and magnesium. Similar supplements are used to increase energy, help relaxation, and reduce cramping and spasms.

PREGNANCY AND CHILDBIRTH: BE EXTRA CAREFUL

Pregnancy is one time when conventional doctors believe in supplementation. We all know that malnutrition has disastrous effects on the development of the fetus. Adequate diet, supplying enough protein, complex carbohydrates, fiber, fresh fruits and vegetables, and essential fatty acids is the first requirement. The second requirement is to avoid toxic chemicals that we know adversely affect the fetus. These chemicals include: most prescription drugs; coffee and any beverage containing caffeine; cigarette smoke; and alcohol.

As for supplementation, we caution you to be prudent about your supplements. Keep in mind that the developing fetus is much more sensitive to biochemical factors than you are. So much growth and development takes place in so short a time, that imbalances that might cause you only minor, temporary discomfort may greatly affect your baby's entire life. It's clear that because a woman plays by different rules when she's pregnant, it's necessary to be more cautious about what kinds and what amounts of supplements she takes.

A good prenatal multivitamin-mineral supplement should supply adequate quantities of all the vitamins and minerals you need. If you have any special supplement needs or wish to take special supplements, however, you should consult your physician before doing so.

ORAL CONTRACEPTIVES
DRAIN NUTRIENTS

We've known for several years that oral contraceptives raise requirements for several vitamins. These include: vitamin A, the B vitamins, vitamin C, vitamin E, and zinc. A woman's need for iron and copper may actually be reduced by oral contraceptives.

It's also possible that combination oral contraceptives increase a woman's risk of cervical cancer. Cervical dysplasia, a precursor of cervical cancer, is much more common in users of oral contraceptives. Folic acid appears to reduce that risk. In high doses, folic acid has been shown to have a beneficial effect on the cervical mucosal surface, reducing or even completely healing abnormal cell growths. It can take several weeks or months for the healing effect to occur. The doses used are in the order of 10 mg. per day. Unfortunately, regulations on the amount of folic acid that can be sold in a single tablet make it difficult to obtain this much of the vitamin. The regulation does not stem from any toxicity of folic acid, but rather from the fact that under rare circumstances, folic acid may mask the existence of B_{12} deficiency.

Beta-carotene is also an important supplement to help prevent cervical cancer. Precancerous cervical dysplasia is more common in women with low blood and dietary levels of beta-carotene. And raising the amount of carotene in the diet has been shown not only to prevent abnormal cell growth on the cervix, but also to reverse it and reestablish a normal cervical environment.

Calcium and magnesium supplements are not only useful in preventing osteoporosis, but also in preventing high blood pressure, another common side effect of the pill. Potassium is also used to prevent high blood pressure.

BREAST CANCER—THE NUTRITIONAL FACTS

How many women know that coffee and other caffeinated beverages can cause the breast lumps in cystic mastitis? We wonder how many women undergo unnecessary biopsies, or experience unnecessary sleepless nights, simply because they've been drinking too much coffee? Although these cysts are not cancerous, there is a higher incidence of breast cancer in women who have these cysts.

Vitamin E supplements can help make the cysts disappear, most likely by normalizing hormone levels. This normalization of hormone levels may also help prevent breast cancer.

Vitamin A supplements may also help. In one study, daily doses of 150,000 I.U. of vitamin A were successful in reducing breast pain and lumps common to benign breast disease, and reducing cancer risk. After six months of taking that much vitamin A, half of the women experienced dry skin and changes in their mucous membranes. We do not recommend taking that much vitamin A for a long period unless you are being carefully monitored by a physician.

Another nutrient that helps protect against breast cancer is selenium. Taken with vitamin E, the protection is greatly enhanced.

Vitamin E, selenium, and vitamin A/ beta-carotene may

also help prevent breast cancer by stimulating the immune system. Also, there is new evidence that EPA (from fish oils) helps prevent breast cancer.

A FINAL WORD ABOUT DIET AND CANCER

Sometimes you not only need to add nutrients to your diet to improve your health and prevent cancer, but you also need to remove some things. To lessen your risk of breast cancer—and also other forms of cancer, especially colon—you should also decrease the amount of fats and oils in your diet. Several studies bear out the fact that as fats in the diet rise, so does the risk of breast and colon cancer.

It's unfortunate that for the past 20 years we have been oversold on the value of polyunsaturated vegetable oils. Although use of these oils may result in lower cholesterol levels than the use of saturated oils or animal fats, they can also result in higher levels of free radicals in the body. The free radicals, in turn, can raise the risk not only of cancer, but also of heart disease. To reduce the risks of both of these diseases, women (and men) should lower their intake of all fats and oils to no more than 30 percent of total caloric intake.

Beyond Vitamins Multisupplement for Women

For additional information on how to design your personal Beyond Vitamins Program, see Chapter 15.

VITAMINS

Vitamin A	20,000 I.U.
Carotene	25,000 I.U.
Thiamine	50–200 mg.

Riboflavin	50–200 mg.
Niacin	50–200 mg.
Pyridoxine	50–200 mg.
Pantothenic acid	100–200 mg.
Folate	400–800 mcg.
B_{12}	100–200 mcg.
Biotin	400 mcg.
Choline	250 mg.
Inositol	100 mg.
Vitamin C	2,000–5,000 mg.
Bioflavonoids	400–1,500 mg.
Vitamin E	400–800 I.U.

MINERALS

Calcium	500–1,500 mg.
Manganese	10–15 mg.
Iron	20 mg.
Magnesium	400–800 mg.
Potassium	100–200 mg.
Selenium	100–200 mcg.
Zinc	20–50 mg.

AMINO ACIDS

Methionine	100 mg.
Cysteine	100 mg.
Glutathione	100 mg.
Tryptophan	500–1,000 mg.
Phenylalanine	500–2,000 mg.

GLANDULARS

Adrenal	50 mg.
Ovarian	50 mg.
Pancreas	50 mg.
Pituitary	50 mg.

ENZYMES

Betaine HCL	100 mg.
Pancreatin	100 mg.
Papain	100 mg.
Bromelain	100 mg.

OTHERS

EPA and/or DHA	500 mg.
GLA	40–240 mg.
DMG	100–200 mg.

PART III

Start Now!

12 How to Begin Your New Multisupplement Program

HOW TO BUY SUPPLEMENTS

Natural versus Synthetic?

One of the oldest and most persistent controversies in nutrition is over whether supplements from natural sources are superior to those from synthetic sources. There should not be controversy at all. In most cases, the issue of natural versus synthetic is used as a marketing tool to claim superiority of a product.

For a start, not all supplements are available in a natural form. The B vitamins and vitamin C are available from natural sources, but not in the amounts we describe in this book. If a B vitamin or vitamin C supplement that supplies more than a few milligrams of any vitamin is called "natural," then you're being sold a product that consists of a few milligrams of natural vitamins, with the bulk of the dose made up from synthetic sources.

Synthetic forms of the B vitamins and vitamin C are fine. There is no reason to doubt the safety or potency of these supplements.

Vitamins A, D, and E are available in natural and synthetic forms in high doses. Vitamins A and D are derived from fish oils, whereas natural vitamin E comes from wheat germ oil, soy, and cottonseed oil. You may want to use both natural and synthetic forms of vitamin A; the natural form is often mixed with vitamin D. If you want to take high doses, however, you will not want to take high doses of vitamin D also. So, you can take most of your dose in a synthetic form and the rest in fish oil.

Natural vitamin E is more potent than synthetic vitamin E. However, the FDA requires that all vitamin E be measured according to potency, so a synthetic vitamin E supplement containing 400 units will have the same potency as a natural 400 unit supplement.

In the case of vitamin D, the natural form is less toxic and, therefore, preferable to the synthetic.

ARE CHELATED MINERALS BETTER?

There are absorption studies which show that the chelated minerals are absorbed better, depending on the chelate used. A chelate is a substance to which the mineral is attached to enhance absorption. Magnesium oxide is an example of a nonchelated mineral. Chelated minerals are called either gluconates, aspartates, citrates, lactates, carbonates, or orotates.

There is some evidence that the gluconates and other, weaker, chelates may not be quite as effective as the aspartates and orotates. The aspartates and orotates are more expensive, however. Our advice is to use them if you have an extreme deficiency and need rapid absorption. But after your body stores are raised, you can switch over to a less-expensive form, such as a gluconate or an oxide.

HOW TO BUY AMINO ACIDS

There are two ways in which amino acid supplements are made. One is by hydrolysis or enzymatic digestion of protein from milk, egg, yeast, soy, or meat. The protein is chemically broken down to make the amino acids more available. There is some predigestion, but the process is not complete. These amino acids may be called "free form," even though they are not truly free form. They will be slightly easier to digest and absorb than if you were to eat a piece of meat, or eggs, or some other protein food.

However, the quality of these protein formulas depends on what amino acids are present. Some of the cheaper protein supplements contain plenty of inexpensive amino acids and smaller quantities of the more expensive ones. Read labels and compare.

True free-form amino acids are synthesized individually. If they appear together, it means they have been mechanically—but not chemically—combined in the tablet. All of the amino acids that are used alone for specific purposes, such as tryptophan, phenylalanine, and carnitine, are synthetic, true free-form amino acids. They are extremely easy to digest. If you have trouble with digestion, of if you're allergic to typical natural sources of hydrolyzed protein supplements, then the synthetic free-form amino acids are for you. Because free-form amino acids are absorbed so quickly, however, if you are taking them to enhance your protein status, take them with meals.

Because they are imported, true free-form amino acids tend to be expensive.

ESSENTIAL OILS ARE ONLY NATURAL

So far, the only good sources of GLA and EPA are totally natural. The vast majority of GLA supplements have been derived from evening primrose oil, to the extent that the two are synonymous. Well, that may be changing. Black currant seed oil, we now know, has more GLA than evening primrose oil. We hope the competition results in lower prices.

EPA is actually present in the oils of just about all wild animals, although it is highest in cold-water fish and cold-weather animals such as seals and polar bears. The vast majority of EPA comes from fish oils.

TIME-RELEASE SUPPLEMENTS
SOMETIMES DON'T!

Many people spend extra money to buy time-release supplements. The rationale behind these is that they will release nutrients into the system over the course of many hours, rather than all at once after a meal.

This is half-science again. First, most supplements taken with meals will be released into the system over the course of several hours, for the simple reason that digestion usually takes from one to four hours.

Second, time-release supplements can actually prevent the release of nutrients at the most opportune times for their absorption and utilization. Studies have shown that these supplements often do not dissolve until they're past the point in the digestive tract where they can be absorbed. And sometimes they do not dissolve at all.

Third, most people do not have a problem digesting too quickly or efficiently—but too slowly and inefficiently.

Taking supplements with your meals will provide you

with the best conditions for absorption and utilization. There is no need to second guess the body.

There is one exception to this rule: vitamin C. Vitamin C is the only nutrient that can be absorbed effectively and reliably when taken in time-release form.

Enteric-coated supplements are also not recommended. The enteric coating is supposed to delay the breakdown of the supplement until it reaches the intestine. Again, studies have shown that the coating can work so well that the tablet never fully breaks down!

HOW TO BUY GLANDULAR SUPPLEMENTS

Glandular supplements are safest and most potent when manufactured by the low-temperature "azeotropic" process, in which an inert, organic solvent is used to remove the fat and other impurities. This process ensures that the enzymes and other potentially active ingredients will be intact and potent.

Some manufacturing processes leave the fat in the gland. This is a bad idea for many reasons. When the fat is left in the glandular supplement, it is subject to oxidation. This produces potentially toxic remnants of rancid fat and very potent free radicals. The fat also contains any pesticide or synthetic hormone residues.

HOW TOXIC ARE YOUR SUPPLEMENTS

In today's world, toxic is a relative term. If you want to be absolute about it, the air we breathe and the water we drink are certifiably toxic. Physicians measure toxicity of a treatment against the danger of withholding the treatment. This is a good standard because it enables one to make a decision. For example, the air may very well contain toxic material, but everyone breathes because not breathing is even more damaging.

Supplements are not absolutely nontoxic. Realistically, however, they are less toxic than the safest over-the-counter medication. They are even safer than most processed foods.

It's extremely difficult to produce a toxic effect with supplements. You have to practically try to do it—over a long period of time. Food supplements are not drugs. They do not affect the body in the same way as drugs. Drugs interfere with or override normal biological reactions, whereas vitamins, minerals, and other food factors are necessary cofactors in them. Nutrients exert their effects by enhancing or facilitating natural body functions.

THE GREAT KIDNEY STONE SCARE

Critics of nutritional supplementation like to say that the preventive and therapeutic use of supplements is hazardous and based on half-truths, incomplete research, and faulty evidence. Actually, the opposite is true. While there is plenty of solid research that supports the benefits of supplements, there is little to support claims that use of supplements is hazardous—and much of what does exist is based on questionable evidence.

The single claim most responsible for scaring people about vitamin C is that taking large doses will raise your urinary oxalate levels and give you kidney stones. Nutritionally-oriented physicians and nutritionists have always known that this claim is false. They've known from their experience that it just doesn't happen. Millions of people have taken billions of grams of vitamin C—and there has been no epidemic of kidney stones.

Now there comes evidence that should silence the kidney stone scare for good. Large doses of vitamin C do not increase either your urinary oxalate levels or your risk of kidney stones. Volunteers were given 8 grams per day of pure vitamin C and their blood and urine levels of oxalate did not increase above presupplementation levels.

There had been experimental evidence that vitamin C did increase oxalate levels. So where did that evidence come from?

It turns out that the prior evidence was based on outmoded lab techniques that gave a false reading. In those prior experiments, oxalate levels were obtained by a method which involved heating the sample. Heating the sample was what caused the high oxalate levels, not the vitamin C; when the sample is not heated, and then tested with modern high-tech methods, there is no increase in oxalate levels. (*European Urology* 9:312-315, 1983).

TAKE SPECIAL CARE

As safe as these Beyond Vitamins multisupplements are, they can also be "strong medicine," and there are certain conditions in which special care should be taken.

- Vitamin A is often cited as an example of a toxic vitamin, but the true toxicity of this nutrient is often exaggerated. Ordinarily, the liver can store up to 1,000,000 units of vitamin A. For the vast majority of people, taking 25,000 units a day for long periods of time should not cause any problems. There are only two or three cases in the scientific literature of doses of 25,000 units or less causing toxicity. Above that daily dose you should be careful. When you get into doses of 100,000 or more, which a physician might use to treat skin conditions or an infection, you're running a higher risk of experiencing symptoms. Such doses should not be taken for more than a week at a time, and always with careful attention to possible symptoms of overdose. Most cases of toxicity reported in the scientific literature are in people taking 100,000 or more units for two months or more.

The first symptoms of vitamin A overdose are persistent headache and blurred vision. Then, as the condition gets worse: chapped lips, dry skin, skin rash, hair that won't wave anymore, joint aches and pains, and a swollen liver, which would cause pain and tenderness in the upper right portion of the belly. Once vitamin A is withdrawn, the symptoms usually go away within two days. Vitamin A toxicity occurs more frequently in people on a low-protein diet.

Realistically, vitamin A toxicity is extremely rare. In my entire career (MR), I have seen only one case. The person had been seeing another doctor, had been taking 100,000 units per day for over two years, and was developing headaches.

There is no danger of vitamin A toxicity from taking carotene. Carotene is converted to vitamin A at a very low rate. A lot of the carotene is used without ever being converted to vitamin A, since carotene has nutritional functions all its own.

• Any B vitamin taken in high doses can cause restlessness and overstimulation. Niacin, in particular, can cause a temporary flush from the release of histamine and prostaglandins. Some people find the flush pleasurable. In any case, it can be reduced by taking a baby aspirin 30 minutes before taking the niacin.

The niacin flush most often happens when the vitamin is taken in the morning, and least after successive doses. After a few weeks of regular use, the flush may stop occurring all by itself. In rare cases, doses of niacin over 100 mg. may cause a persistent skin rash.

Niacin also raises blood sugar and so should be used with caution by diabetics. It can raise uric acid levels and so should be used with caution in people with gout. Niacin can also raise hydrochloric acid levels and so should be used with caution by people with ulcers.

• Pyridoxine, or B$_6$, is generally safe. There have been some isolated cases reported in the scientific literature of pyridoxine overdose causing "sensory neuropathy," or "pins and needles" sensations, loss of balance and coordination, wobbling gait, and possible destruction of cells in the spinal cord. In these reports, between 2,000 and 5,000 mg. of pyridoxine were being used— without corresponding doses of the other B-complex vitamins. Other B vitamins, especially riboflavin, are required for the proper utilization of pyridoxine. When an extremely high dose of pyridoxine is given without accompanying doses of the other B vitamins, an acute riboflavin deficiency can develop, which is apparently what happened in these cases.

In this book, we do not recommend taking more than 200 mg. of pyridoxine per day, unless you are under a physician's care. There have been many controlled studies which have found no adverse effects at doses as high as 200 mg. We do not recommend taking *any* pyridoxine without accompanying doses of other B vitamins.

Nevertheless, if you're taking pyridoxine and experiencing pins and needles sensations, difficulty in your manual coordination, or burning in your feet and toes, you may be taking too much. If toxicity symptoms occur, they may take weeks or months to dissipate.

• High doses of vitamin C will occasionally cause stomach upset, bloating, gas, flatulence, and/or diarrhea. This reaction is not, in itself, dangerous. We interpret it as a sign that you are taking more vitamin C than your body needs and wants to absorb at the moment. Just reduce the dose or switch to calcium ascorbate or sodium ascorbate.

• Vitamin D in extremely high doses can cause calcium to be deposited in the wrong places. The dose we recommend in this book is safe, but vitamin D should be used with caution by anyone with gallstones or kidney stones.

- Calcium should be used with caution by people with gallstones or kidney stones. Your dose should be managed by your personal physician.
- Vitamin E can lower thyroid hormone activity. If you're taking thyroid hormone and vitamin E and notice that you feel more fatigued or that your need for thyroid hormone is raised, then you may be taking too much vitamin E. Generally, this effect will not take place at or below 400 units per day.
- Iodine at a dose of 100 to 200 mcg. per day should be safe. At very high doses, iodine can promote acne. There is also evidence that thyroiditis (Hashimoto's), which afflicts about 6 percent of women, may be made worse by iodine. Be aware that iodine is present in iodized salt and seaweed products.
- In high doses, potassium can cause problems for persons with serious kidney or heart disease.
- Zinc should be safe at the doses recommended in this book. At very high doses, zinc can lower body stores of copper and manganese, and raise cholesterol levels. Someone with high cholesterol levels should not take more than 100 mg. of zinc per day.

  With mineral supplements, the body protects itself by adjusting absorption to fit its requirements. Nevertheless, dose recommendations should not be exceeded. Trace minerals, especially, are effective over a relatively narrow range of doses. Zinc is perhaps the most important supplement for the immune system. However, excessive doses of zinc may suppress certain functions of the immune system. Do not take more than 100 mg. of zinc daily, unless a higher dose is recommended by your personal physician.

- Lysine will not work well if you're also taking arginine or eating a high-arginine diet (nuts and seeds.)
- Phenylalanine and tyrosine in high doses can raise adrenalin levels, make you nervous, and cause rapid heart beat. This effect can be exacerbated by caffeine and nasal decongestants.

- In high doses, tryptophan can cause sedation.
- Histidine and cysteine can interfere with zinc absorption and reduce zinc levels. It is best to take these amino acids at a different time than when zinc supplements are taken.
- HCL supplements can cause burning in the stomach and should not be used by persons with ulcers.
- In very high doses (exceeding six capsules per day), EPA or fish oils can severely reduce the blood's ability to clot. The Eskimos, who consume vast quantities of these oils, often get bloody noses and bruise easily. If a person is already on blood-thinning drugs, these supplements should be taken only under a doctor's supervision. Keep in mind that even one capsule can somewhat reduce the blood's clotting ability.
- Pregnant women should not undertake any supplementation program without consulting their physician. Amino acid supplements should not be taken by a pregnant or lactating woman unless her personal physician advises it.
- Persons under a physician's care and taking prescription drugs for any chronic condition should not reduce or discontinue their medication without consulting their personal physician.
- If you have any condition, genetic or otherwise, that may interfere with the utilization of amino acids (such as phenylketonuria, a genetic inability to metabolize phenylalanine), do not take amino acid supplements without consulting your personal physician.
- Persons receiving medication for Parkinson's disease should not take B vitamin supplements without consulting their physician. Pyridoxine, or B_6, can interfere with the drug L-dopa.
- If you have high blood pressure or rheumatic heart disease, do not take vitamin E or phenylalanine without first consulting your doctor. These supplements can raise blood pressure in susceptible individuals.
- Persons with kidney disease or stomach ulcers should

not take supplements without first consulting their physician.

- Follow this principle when taking supplements, a principle that nutritionally-trained physicians use: Always start with the lowest doses and gradually increase doses until you achieve the desired effect. Don't expect immediate results in all cases. Supplements generally do not work by immediately interfering in bodily functions. Rather, they gently stimulate or normalize metabolic activity. This can take time, so be patient.
- Allergy to essential nutrients is highly unlikely. However, allergies to the materials from which the nutrients are derived, or to the tableting materials, is common. If you experience an allergic reaction to a supplement, try to find out the source of the nutrient and the materials used in constructing the tablet. Then switch to a "hypo-allergenic" supplement or one that does not contain materials to which you are allergic.
- If you experience any adverse effects, discontinue your supplements and consult a nutritionally-trained physician.

Finally, a book can go only so far in describing the best supplement plans for supporting and boosting your health. The science of nutritional therapy has made some great advances within the past few years. Nutritionally-trained physicians now have accurate laboratory tests which can almost pinpoint your needs for essential and therapeutic nutrients. We believe that the programs in this book will help the vast majority of people use supplements to their best advantage. Nevertheless, please do not hesitate to take advantage of the new advances in nutritional diagnosis should the need arise.

13 Seven Nutrition Tips That Can Make a Difference in How Well Your Supplements Work

1. DRINK WATER WITH YOUR MEALS

There is a myth whose time has come—to be put to rest for good. The myth is: Don't drink water with your meals because you'll dilute your digestive enzymes. This myth is all wet!

A cup of water with your meal will boost digestive efficiency, not diminish it. We know it seems scientific to say that the water will dilute everything. But that's only half-science.

Water is the universal solvent. It helps dissolve the food and actually stimulates acid secretion. Don't worry about your food or your supplements being "washed away through the digestive tract and out of the body." The body doesn't work that way. The digestive system is not passive plumbing, but rather a series of very active organs and glands.

2. TAKE YOUR SUPPLEMENTS WITH YOUR MEALS

Vitamins can be absorbed on an empty stomach, and for some supplements, such as the amino acid tryptophan, it's necessary to aid in selective uptake. However, the best time to take most of your supplements is at mealtime—preferably during or immediately after the meal.

Supplements are concentrated food substances. In order for them to be absorbed and utilized to their maximum potential, they should be digested along with your food. They need the action of the various digestive enzymes, which will not be fully secreted if you take the supplements between meals.

Also, many of the supplements play their most important roles as supporting actors to the nutrients in your food. The B vitamins, for example, aid in carbohydrate, fat, and protein metabolism. Doesn't it make sense that it helps if there is some carbohydrate, fat, and protein there for them to help metabolize?

Finally, when you take your supplements between meals, you increase the chances of causing an upset stomach or nausea.

3. AVOID POLYUNSATURATED OILS

Despite what the margarine and salad oil commercials say, polyunsaturated oils are not as friendly as we once thought they were. Here's why:

Free radicals, as you by now know, can be major villains as far as our health is concerned (see Chapter 6). A prime source of free radicals is the oxidation of oils, lipids—or fatty acids—in the body. Not only do fatty acids circulate in the blood, but they also make up important structural parts of every cell.

Now, the body needs a certain amount of unsaturated fatty acids. The essential fatty acids must be supplied in the diet. But remember: Though all essential fatty acids are unsaturated, not all unsaturated oils are essential, or even beneficial. Unfortunately, polyunsaturated oils are not only a major source of essential fatty acids, but also a major source of free radicals.

Because they contain so many unsaturated fat molecules, these oils are very unstable and ripe for oxidation. They're like the proverbial accident waiting to happen. Just sitting at room temperature, they are constantly being oxidized, generating free radicals. When they're heated, they become even more unstable.

Polyunsaturated oils in high amounts also suppress the immune system. We don't know exactly how this occurs, but we do know that certain polyunsaturated oils stimulate the production of inflammatory prostaglandins, which also suppress the immune system.

The combination of their immune-suppressing and free radical-producing effects may help explain why increased use of polyunsaturated oils is suspected of promoting cancer and heart disease.

Not all vegetable oils are polyunsaturated. Olive oil and peanut oil are monounsaturated and far more stable than polyunsaturated oils. They are also more stable when heated.

Our recommendation is to minimize the use of all oils in the diet, but to use olive oil instead of other vegetable oils. Artificially hydrogenated oils, such as are found in margarine and other processed foods, are to be totally avoided. They are even worse than polyunsaturated oils! Processed, hardened oils and margarines contain "trans fatty acids," which—in addition to all the above nutritional crimes—can also interfere with essential fatty acid metabolism and cause a deficiency.

4. CABBAGE JUICE CAN HEAL ULCERS

This may seem like a joke, but to thousands of people suffering from ulcers, this information has been a godsend. It's also a fascinating story of how circumstances can combine to take a treatment that is on the brink of revolutionizing standard medical care for a disease—and turn it into the one of the most well-kept secrets on earth.

First, the secret: Raw cabbage juice, administered two or three times a day, can relieve pain from ulcers and immediately and drastically reduce the time required for healing. This treatment was researched, developed, and tested by Dr. Garnett Cheney in the 1940s. His work began with animals and culminated in a controlled, double-blind experiment in which the effects of cabbage juice were tested against the effects of a placebo. Dr. Cheney's results were consistent. Cabbage juice always reduced pain and sped up the healing process.

So why didn't cabbage juice become the standard treatment for ulcers? Was it a conspiracy on the part of the FDA and the drug companies?

No. Actually, much of Dr. Cheney's work was supported by a major drug company, in hopes of identifying the active ingredient in the cabbage juice. For a while, this "mystery ingredient" was called vitamin U.

What happened was a series of mostly unconnected incidents, which combined to effectively scuttle the use of cabbage juice—at least in the United States. First, Dr. Cheney died before his last study was completed. His co-workers faithfully carried out and reported the results of the experiment. But no one took up the fallen banner to champion Dr. Cheney's work.

Second, the drug company chemists could never isolate and identify the active ingredient in the cabbage juice. Their interest was, of course, in synthesizing it and manufacturing it in mass quantities. Understandably, they were not interested in getting into the juice business.

The final blow was dealt by historical advances in the science of drugs. Right around the time when the drug companies were running into frustrations with cabbage juice, they made incredible breakthroughs in the development of steroid drugs. Suddenly, all the scientific interest was diverted to steroid drugs, which were rightly considered extremely important, as well as profitable. Research into why cabbage juice heals ulcers was abandoned—in the United States, anyway.

Other countries, notably Great Britain, Russia, and Hungary, have continued testing cabbage juice on ulcers—and have continued to document its effectiveness. We now know that the active healing ingredient in cabbage juice is allantoin, which also happens to be present in aloe vera and comfrey leaf. I (MR) have had many patients whose ulcers have healed rapidly, sometimes within a few days, when taking aloe vera juice. It tastes very bitter and can be diluted with water or juice. (Aloe vera juice is also effective at helping burns to heal, when applied directly to the burn.)

5. ATHLETES NEED MORE ANTIOXIDANTS

We've seen the debate in sports and fitness magazines time after time: Do athletes and people who exercise a lot need extra supplements? Do they need supplements at all?

The answer is yes. And the reason is very simple. Exercise—especially aerobic exercise—generates lots of damaging free radicals. When you exercise, you pump oxygen through your body at a higher, faster rate. Your body's going to need all the help it can get to scavenge up all those free radicals before they cause damage. So, at the very least, exercising people should take supplements of antioxidants.

Most professional and world class athletes don't have to be told to take supplements. They do it because they know it helps their performance. It's the "neighborhood-class" athletes and the weekend warriors who need to know this fact. We've never seen this revealed in the exercise and sports magazines—so now that you know, tell a friend.

6. DON'T TAKE YOUR MINERALS AND BRAN AT THE SAME MEAL

Along with all the wonderful things bran—oat, wheat, corn, or whatever kind—does, it can also cause you to waste money on mineral supplements. Here's how: bran— actually all fiber, especially fiber from grains—contains chemicals called phytates, which can bind with minerals and prevent their absorption. Zinc is especially vulnerable to inhibition of absorption by phytates in whole grains.

Because of this, we shudder when we see people taking their mineral supplements after a wonderful breakfast of whole grain cereal and extra bran!

So . . . do not take your mineral supplements at the same meals at which you either eat a lot of whole grains or use extra bran. Plan one meal a day where you will not use extra bran or lots of grains—and then take your mineral supplements.

7. ONE LAST SUPPLEMENT . . .

This is a "supplement" we're taught about in grammar school—but forget by the time we're in high school. It's one supplement that can, by itself, greatly increase the amount of nutrients we absorb and utilize.

It's one supplement, however, that doesn't come in a bottle: chewing.

If you supplement each one of your meals with about 50 percent more chewing before you swallow, you will greatly increase the nutrients you absorb. We learn in grammar school that digestion begins in the mouth, but so many of us forget and fail to take advantage of our own digestive standard equipment.

The advantage of extra chewing is that it breaks up food particles and gives your enzymes more surface area to work on, thus increasing the efficiency of digestion.

CHAPTER

14 The Ultimate Nutrition Secret

THE LAST nutrition secret is one we can't reveal in this book. No book can, because the last secret is YOU. Only you can unlock the secrets of your own needs and desires. Only you can decide whether or not you want the benefits of Beyond Vitamins supplements. Only you can decide which supplements to take, and only you can monitor your own feelings and responses in order to tell how much you need of each nutrient. You're in complete charge.

And that's the way it should be.

You see, taking supplements is not passive. The people we know who take supplements are not passive sorts who like to be told what to do. They began to take supplements as part of a beginning effort to play a more active role in building and maintaining their own health.

LET YOUR SUPER LIFE BEGIN HERE

Notice, we said a "beginning" effort. They all went on to add other activities to their personal health and fitness programs. And you should, too.

Your committment to living a super life should not end with taking supplements. Supplements are just what the word implies—they are things which are to be added.

Added to what? To your total commitment, to everything you do to boost yourself beyond the ordinary, beyond the level of health and fitness that too many people are satisfied with.

We've written this book as a first step for everyone to take beyond vitamins and beyond ordinary energy, vigor, susceptibility to disease . . . beyond ordinary mental, physical, and sexual performance. The next steps are up to you. This is the secret that only you can reveal.

These are exciting times we live in, especially for people who want to find out all they can about how nutrition can help us live the super life. We are living in the middle of a veritable explosion of information about nutrition and fitness. In this book, we've brought you one important part of that nutritional cutting edge. We hope you'll take advantage of this information and begin to take your next steps today.

CHAPTER

15 The Beyond
Vitamins Workbook

THIS IS the part of the book in which you will design your own personal Beyond Vitamins multisupplement. The steps are simple to follow. In no time at all you will know what to take and how much to take in order to nutritionally support the benefits we've been discussing in all of the previous chapters.

1. Look at the Dose Range Chart on pages 202–205 and mark or circle the columns that correspond to the specific fitness benefits that you want. Be sure to circle the Basic, because that one ensures that you're getting all the basic vitamins and minerals, plus a few other important fundamental supplements. If you're also interested in boosting your immune system, for example, mark that column. If you're on a weight loss diet, plus you want maximum performance, then mark those two columns, and so on.

2. After you've marked all the columns you want, then read across each line and find and mark the lowest dose of each supplement that appears on that line. Write that low dose in the space for that supplement in Your Personal Multisupplement Chart on pages 206–208. You may not be writing down a dose for every supplement. For example, if you marked the columns for Basic, Immunity, and Women, you will circle the low dose for vitamin A at 10,000 I.U.

3. Now circle the highest dose for each supplement and write it in the space provided in Your Personal Multisupplement Chart. For example, if you marked the columns for Basic, Immunity, and Women, you will circle and write 20,000 I.U. as your high dose for vitamin A.

4. You now have your low dose and high dose for every supplement that is part of your Beyond Vitamins Personal Multisupplement.

HOW TO BEGIN YOUR NEW SUPPLEMENT PROGRAM A LITTLE AT A TIME

People adjust to taking supplements more easily if they introduce new supplements a few at a time rather than all at once. The Beyond Vitamins Workbook will allow you to introduce your new supplements over a period of seven weeks. Weekly Planners on pages 208–210 headlined "Week One, Week Two," and so on will help you design your supplement program. You will record your dose ranges in the blank spaces for each week, according to what fitness or therapeutic benefits you identify on the dose range chart. Then you will be ready to use the supplements in the following order:

Week One: Begin with the vitamins, minerals, and bio-flavonoids.
Week Two: Add enzymes.
Week Three: Add amino acids.
Week Four: Add oils.
Week Five: Add DMG.
Week Six: Add mucopolysaccharides.
Week Seven: Add glandulars.

HOW TO GO FROM THE LOW DOSE TO THE HIGH DOSE

If you were under the care of a nutritionally trained physician, you would be able to undergo many sophisticated tests to determine your immune competence, your blood and tissue levels of certain nutrients, your amino acid and mineral balances, and other aspects of your nutritional health. For someone who is ill, there is no substitute for this kind of sophisticated care of a physician.

Even under the care of a physician using the most advanced nutritional status tests, however, the most important guiding principle in deciding what to take and how much is still how you feel. Whether or not your nutritional program is helping you feel better is more important than how it's affecting your test results. And you don't need test results to know how you're feeling.

So the first principle in deciding how, when, and by how much to raise your supplement doses is to be aware of how your supplements are affecting you. The second principle is that you are going to start at the low dose of every nutrient and slowly increase the dose, if you so wish.

Well, you ask, how long should you wait until you go on to a higher dose?

There is no definite answer to that question. With some supplements, such as enzymes, some of the amino acids, vitamin C, and the B vitamins, you may notice a change within a day or two. With minerals the effects may take a month or more, until body stores are built up. With the fat-soluble vitamins and the essential oils, the effects may take several weeks or even months.

For the purpose of establishing a guideline, we are going to ask you to wait at least two weeks before raising your doses. If you do not notice any beneficial effects within two weeks of taking a supplement, raise the dose slightly. Each time you raise the dose, raise it by approximately one-fourth to one-third the original dose, until you feel a benefit or reach the maximum dose in the range. We also believe it is a good idea to back off from higher doses once your special needs are met. Once you're feeling better, you may want to work your way down to the basic doses.

If you notice any adverse effects, then stop taking the supplement immediately. Wait two weeks after the symptoms have gone away, and then, if you wish, begin to take the supplement again—but at half the original dose. In pages 181–186 we give you complete information about potential adverse effects.

IF YOU DON'T WANT TO TAKE ALL OF YOUR SUPPLEMENTS ALL OF THE TIME

Please don't interpret the plan your Workbook comes up with as the *only* way to take these supplements. Once you are taking a basic vitamin-mineral supplement, you can use the Beyond Vitamins supplement individually or in combinations for the nutritional purposes described in the chapters. For example, you may want to take carnitine just for a few weeks or months, while on a diet or while in training. Or you might decide to take some enzymes and bioflavonoids, with vitamin C, for a day or two in order to relieve some inflammation from an athletic strain.

Remember, our recommendations can be taken as a complete program, or as a "bible" of complete information, from which you pick and choose according to your own needs and desires.

HOW TO TAKE YOUR SUPPLEMENTS

Most supplements should be taken with or after your meals. Only a few can or should be taken on an empty stomach.

High doses can be divided up so that you take them two

or three times a day. This is a problem for many people, however, so don't feel it is absolutely necessary to do it this way. It will give you a slight increase in absorption efficiency. But you don't want to do that at the expense of making your supplement program a nuisance.

Vitamin C can be taken on an empty stomach. If you take it that way, you can achieve a higher absorption faster, which might be desirable if you're fighting off an infection. If you take it with a meal, however, the vitamin will be absorbed more slowly. Ultimately, more of it will be absorbed that way. We find ourselves taking it both ways.

Free-form amino acids, if taken as general protein supplements, should be taken with meals to maximize utilization.

Certain amino acids must be taken alone, on an empty stomach, to ensure absorption and proper utilization. These include tryptophan, phenylalanine, and tyrosine. These three should not be taken together with one another, nor with meals or any other amino acid supplement. If you need to take all three, take tryptophan at night before bed, and in the morning before breakfast; take phenylalanine or tyrosine between meals. Lysine should also be taken before breakfast, so put off your tryptophan until evening.

Taking enzymes or certain glandular extracts such as pancreatic extract may enhance absorption of vitamins and minerals.

Many people take fiber supplements or add extra bran to one or more meals during the day. Because substances in bran can interfere with absorption of minerals, we recommend that you do not take your mineral supplements with high-fiber meals.

THINKING FOR YOURSELF

People who take supplements are often criticized as the victims of ignorance, which leaves them susceptible to a massive conspiracy to swindle and prevent them from seeking adequate diet or medical care. This, too, is non-sense. Demographic studies of people who take supplements have demonstrated that they are among the most highly educated segments of society. The know a lot about nutrition, fitness, and health, and apply their knowledge in all aspects of their diet and life, not just supplementation.

Do people who take supplements neglect other areas of their diet? Not in the least!

We know from experience that taking supplements is often the first of many steps taken to adopt better diet and health habits. By taking supplements, you are making a visible sign to yourself and to the world that you care enough about your health and fitness to take this extra step. You are, in effect, saying to yourself, *"I can make a difference in my health and strength and happiness."*

Do you know what a powerful statement that is? We've seen it revolutionize people's lives—beginning with our own.

We hope it's a statement you'll make too.

Beyond Vitamins Dose Range Chart

VITAMINS	Basic (Chapter 3)	Stress (Chapter 4)	Immunity (Chapter 5)	Youth Extension (Chapter 6)
Vitamin A	10,000 I.U.	10,000 I.U.	25,000 I.U.	10,000 I.U.
Carotene	20,000 I.U.	25,000 I.U.	25,000 I.U.	25,000 I.U.
Thiamine	50 mg.	50 mg.		50 mg.
Riboflavin	50 mg.	50 mg.		50 mg.
Niacin	50 mg.	50–200 mg.		50 mg.
Pyridoxine	50 mg.	50 mg.	50 mg.	50 mg.
Pantothenic acid	100 mg.	100–1,000 mg.	100–1,000 mg.	100 mg.
Folic acid	400 mcg.	400 mcg.	800–2,000 mcg.	400 mcg.
B$_{12}$	100 mcg.	100 mcg.		100 mcg.
Biotin	400 mcg.	400 mcg.		400 mcg.
Choline	250 mcg.	250 mcg.		500 mg.
Inositol	100 mg.	100 mg.		100–250 mg.
PABA	100 mg.	100 mg.		
Vitamin C	1,000 mg.	1,000–10,000 mg.	2,000–10,000 mg.	1,000–5,000 mg
Bioflavonoids	200 mg.	200–1,000 mg.	1,000–2,000 mg.	500 mg.
Vitamin D	200 I.U.			
Vitamin E	200 I.U.	200–400 I.U.	400–800 I.U.	200–600 I.U.

MINERALS	Basic (Chapter 3)	Stress (Chapter 4)	Immunity (Chapter 5)	Youth Extension (Chapter 6)
Calcium	500 mg.	500–1,000 mg.		500–1,500 mg.
Chromium	100 mcg.	200 mcg.		100 mcg.
Iodine	100 mcg.			
Iron				
Magnesium	250 mg.	250–500 mg.		250 mg.
Manganese	10 mg.			10 mg.
Molybdenum	50 mcg.			
Potassium	100 mg.	200 mg.		
Selenium	100 mcg.	100–200 mcg.	100–200 mcg.	100 mcg.
Silicon	100 mg.			
Zinc	30 mg.	50 mg.	30–100 mg.	30–50 mg.

ENZYMES	Basic (Chapter 3)	Stress (Chapter 4)	Immunity (Chapter 5)	Youth Extension (Chapter 6)
Betaine HCL				100 mg.
Pancreatin				100 mg.
Papain			100 mg.	100 mg.
Bromelain		100–500 mg.	100 mg.	100 mg.
Pepsin			100 mg.	
Bile factors				100 mg.

Performance (Chapter 7)	Weight Loss (Chapter 8)	Sex (Chapter 9)	Allergies (Chapter 10)	Women (Chapter 11)
10,000 I.U.	10,000 I.U.	10,000 I.U.	10,000–20,000 I.U.	20,000 I.U.
25,000–50,000 I.U.		25,000 I.U.	25,000 I.U.	25,000 I.U.
100 mg.	50 mg.	50 mg.	50 mg.	50–200 mg.
100 mg.	50 mg.	50 mg.	50 mg.	50–200 mg.
100–500 mg.	50 mg.	50 mg.	50–500 mg.	50–200 mg.
100 mg.	50 mg.	50 mg.	50 mg.	50–200 mg.
100–500 mg.	100 mg.	100–300 mg.	100–500 mg.	100–200 mg.
400 mcg.	400 mcg.	400 mcg.	400 mcg.	400–800 mcg.
100 mcg.	100 mcg.	100 mcg.	100 mcg.	100–200 mcg.
400 mcg.	400 mcg.	400 mcg.	400 mcg.	400 mcg.
1,000–10,000 mg. (P)	250 mg.	250 mg.	250 mg.	250 mg.
100 mg.	100 mg.	100–200 mg.	100 mg.	100 mg.
100 mg.	100 mg.	100 mg.	100 mg.	
4,000–8,000 mg.	1,000–4,000 mg.	1,000–3,000 mg.	2,000–8,000 mg.	2,000–5,000 mg.
500–2,000 mg.	200–1,000 mg.	200–1,000 mg.	500–4,000 mg.	400–1,500 mg.
400–800 I.U.	100–400 I.U.	200–600 I.U.	200–400 I.U.	400–800 I.U.

Performance (Chapter 7)	Weight Loss (Chapter 8)	Sex (Chapter 9)	Allergies (Chapter 10)	Women (Chapter 11)
500 mg.	500–1,000 mg.	500 mg.		500–1,500 mg.
200–500 mcg.	200 mcg.			
100 mcg.				
				20 mg.
250 mg.	250–500 mg.	400 mg.		400–800 mg.
10–15 mg.	10 mg.			10–15 mg.
100–200 mg.	100 mg.	100 mg.		100–200 mg.
200 mcg.		100–200 mcg.		100–200 mcg.
30 mg.		15–100 mg.	30–75 mg.	20–50 mg.

Performance (Chapter 7)	Weight Loss (Chapter 8)	Sex (Chapter 9)	Allergies (Chapter 10)	Women (Chapter 11)
100 mg.	100 mg.		100 mg.	100 mg.
100 mg.	100 mg.		100 mg.	100 mg.
100–500 mg.			100 mg.	100 mg.
100–500 mg.			100 mg.	100 mg.
	100 mg.		100 mg.	

AMINO ACIDS	Basic (Chapter 3)	Stress (Chapter 4)	Immunity (Chapter 5)	Youth Extension (Chapter 6)
Glutamine				Free-form
Carnitine		100 mg.		supplement
Cystine				supplying
Lysine			1,000 mg. (BB)	most AA in
Methionine		100 mg.		varying
Cysteine		100 mg.		amounts)
Glutathione		200–500 mg.	200 mg.	
Leucine				
Isoleucine				
Ornithine			1,000–2,000 mg.	
Arginine		100 mg.	1,000–3,000 mg.	
Taurine		100 mg.	100–500 mg.	
Glycine		100 mg.		
Tyrosine		200–500 mg.		1,000 mg.
Tryptophan				500–1,500 mg
Phenylalanine		200–500 mg.		1,000 mg.
Glutamic acid		100 mg.		
Valine				
Alanine				
Aspartic acid				
Histidine				

*Plus a free-form amino acid supplement

GLANDULARS	Basic (Chapter 3)	Stress (Chapter 4)	Immunity (Chapter 5)	Youth Extension (Chapter 6)
Adrenal		50–600 mg.	50 mg.	50 mg.
Testicular				50 mg.
Ovarian				50 mg.
Pancreas				50 mg.
Thymus			50 mg.	50 mg.
Thyroid			50 mg.	50 mg.
Stomach				50 mg.
Duodenum				50 mg.
Liver		50–3,000 mg.		500 mg.
Heart				50 mg.
Pituitary				50 mg.
Spleen			50 mg.	50 mg.
Brain				50 mg.

OTHERS	Basic (Chapter 3)	Stress (Chapter 4)	Immunity (Chapter 5)	Youth Extension (Chapter 6)
EPA (fish oil)		500–1,000 mg.		500 mg.
GLA (EPO)		40 mg. (500 mg.)	40 mg. (500 mg.)	
Germanium			100 mg.	
Octacosanol				
Mucopolysaccharides		200 mg.		200 mg.
DMG		100–200 mg.	100–200 mg.	

Performance* (Chapter 7)	Weight Loss (Chapter 8)	Sex (Chapter 9)	Allergies (Chapter 10)	Women (Chapter 11)
	100–1,000 mg.			
500–5,000 mg.	500–4,000 mg.			
	100 mg.			
500–3,000 mg.				
100–500 mg.	100 mg.		100 mg.	100 mg.
			100 mg.	100 mg.
100–500 mg.	100–250 mg.		100 mg.	100 mg.
100–1,000 mg.	100–500 mg.			
100–1,000 mg.	100–500 mg.			
500–1,000 mg.				
500–1,000 mg.				
	100–500 mg.			
100–1,000 mg.		100–250 mg.		
500–2,000 mg.		100–500 mg.	500–1,000 mg.	
500–2,000 mg.	500–1,500 mg.	500–1,500 mg.		500–1,000 mg.
500–2,000 mg.	500–1,000 mg.	500–1,500 mg.		500–2,000 mg.
100–1,000 mg.		100–250 mg.		
100–1,000 mg.	100–500 mg.			
		100–250 mg.		
500–1,000 mg.				
			100 mg.	

Performance (Chapter 7)	Weight Loss (Chapter 8)	Sex (Chapter 9)	Allergies (Chapter 10)	Women (Chapter 11)
50 mg.	50 mg.	50 mg.	50–500 mg.	50 mg.
		50 mg.		
		50 mg.		50 mg.
50 mg.	50 mg.		50 mg.	50 mg.
			50 mg.	
		50 mg.		
	50 mg.		50 mg.	
	50 mg.		50 mg.	
500 mg.	500 mg.		500 mg.	
50 mg.				
		50 mg.		50 mg.

Performance (Chapter 7)	Weight Loss (Chapter 8)	Sex (Chapter 9)	Allergies (Chapter 10)	Women (Chapter 11)
500–1,000 mg.		500 mg.	500 mg.	500 mg.
	50–250 mg.	40 mg. (500 mg.)	40–240 mg. (500 mg.)	40–240 mg. (500 mg.)
250 mcg.	250 mcg.			
200 mg.		100–200 mg.	100 mg.	
100–200 mg.	100–200 mg.		100 mg.	100–240 mg.

Your Personal Multisupplement Chart

VITAMINS	LOW DOSE	HIGH DOSE
Vitamin A		
Carotene		
Thiamine		
Riboflavin		
Niacin		
Pyridoxine		
Pantothenic acid		
Folic acid		
B_{12}		
Biotin		
Choline		
Inositol		
PABA		
Vitamin C		
Bioflavonoids		
Vitamin D		
Vitamin E		

MINERALS	LOW DOSE	HIGH DOSE
Calcium		
Chromium		
Iodine		
Iron		
Magnesium		
Manganese		
Molybdenum		
Potassium		
Selenium		
Silicon		
Zinc		

ENZYMES	LOW DOSE	HIGH DOSE
Betaine HCL		
Pancreatin		
Papain		
Bromelain		
Pepsin		
Bile factors		

AMINO ACIDS	LOW DOSE	HIGH DOSE
Glutamine		
Carnitine		
Cystine		
Lysine		
Methionine		
Cysteine		
Glutathione		
Leucine		
Isoleucine		
Ornithine		
Arginine		
Taurine		
Glycine		
Tyrosine		
Tryptophan		
Phenylalanine		
Glutamic acid		
Valine		
Alanine		
Aspartic acid		
Histidine		

GLANDULARS	LOW DOSE	HIGH DOSE
Adrenal		
Testicular		
Ovarian		
Pancreas		
Thymus		
Thyroid		
Stomach		
Duodenum		
Liver		
Heart		
Pituitary		
Spleen		
Brain		

Your Personal Multisupplement Chart (*cont.*)

OTHERS	LOW DOSE	HIGH DOSE
EPA (fish oil)	___	___
GLA (EPO)	___	___
Germanium	___	___
Octacosanol	___	___
Mucopolysaccharides	___	___
DMG	___	___

Your Weekly Planners

Week One: Build Your Foundation

VITAMINS	DOSE
Vitamin A	___
Carotene	___
Thiamine	___
Riboflavin	___
Niacin	___
Pyridoxine	___
Pantothenic acid	___
Folic acid	___
B_{12}	___
Biotin	___
Choline	___
Inositol	___
PABA	___
Vitamin C	___
Bioflavonoids	___
Vitamin D	___
Vitamin E	___

MINERALS	DOSE
Calcium	___
Chromium	___
Iodine	___
Iron	___

Magnesium _____
Manganese _____
Molybdenum _____
Potassium _____
Selenium _____
Silicon _____
Zinc _____

Week Two: Add Enzymes

DOSE

Betaine HCL _____
Pancreatin _____
Papain _____
Bromelain _____
Pepsin _____
Bile factors _____

Week Three: Add Amino Acids

DOSE

Glutamine _____
Carnitine _____
Cystine _____
Lysine _____
Methionine _____
Cysteine _____
Glutathione _____
Leucine _____
Isoleucine _____
Ornithine _____
Arginine _____
Taurine _____
Glycine _____
Tyrosine _____
Tryptophan _____
Phenylalanine _____
Glutamic acid _____
Valine _____
Alanine _____
Aspartic acid _____
Histidine _____

Your Weekly Planners (*cont.*)

Week Four: Add Oils

	DOSE
EPA (fish oil)	_____
GLA (EPO)	_____

Week Five: Add DMG

	DOSE
DMG	_____

Week Six: Add Mucopolysaccharides

	DOSE
Mucopolysaccharides	_____

Week Seven: Add Glandulars

	DOSE
Adrenal	_____
Testicular	_____
Ovarian	_____
Pancreas	_____
Thymus	_____
Thyroid	_____
Stomach	_____
Duodenum	_____
Liver	_____
Heart	_____
Pituitary	_____
Spleen	_____
Brain	_____

APPENDIX A
A Beyond Vitamins Primer
Basic Information about Vitamins, Minerals and Other Supplements

VITAMINS

Vitamin A—Our Guardian

Think of vitamin A as a kind of "palace guard" for our body: It takes care of the barriers and openings to the outside world. If we have enough vitamin A, our eyes will be clear and bright and our bones and teeth strong. Our skin will be moist and youthful. Vitamin A keeps the mucous membranes in top working order. Maybe you never stopped to think about your mucous membranes, but they are your first line of defense against any unwanted organism or substance that wants to enter the vulnerable interior of your body.

Vitamin A maintains the adrenal glands, which are crucial if we want to respond in the appropriate manner to all kinds of stimuli—from stress to sex.

Vitamin A helps us guard against infections through its direct stimulation of the immune system. In this regard, vitamin A is unique, because it offers nonspecific immune protection—it stimulates the immune system's battles against all intruders. Vitamin A also boosts immunity by maintaining the mucous membranes and boosting the production of mucus, which acts as a lubricant for sensitive membranes and as a trap for invading organisms.

Vitamin A also helps us heal faster, helps control heavy menstrual bleeding, and has been found to be a factor in preventing some forms of cancer, specifically oral and cervical. Vitamin A prevents and reverses mouth cancer caused by chewing tobacco, and it prevents and reverses abnormal PAP smears.

THE SUPER NUTRIENT THAT WAS HIDING BEHIND VITAMIN A

Carotene was once thought of only as a precursor of vitamin A, but now we know it's much, much more. As a precursor, carotene is converted to vitamin A by the body. But not all the carotene is converted to vitamin A, and that which remains is important in its own right. Carotene is a powerful antioxidant, similar to vitamin E in that it protects the vulnerable lipid, or fatty, layer of the cell.

Also, carotene has been found to help prevent several forms of cancer, including cancer of the breast, skin, mouth, cervix, lung, colon, gastrointestinal tract, and bladder. Studies have shown that people with higher levels of beta-carotene in their diets have less risk of developing these forms of cancer.

Studies have also shown that women with diets high in beta-carotene and vitamin C have less risk of developing cervical cancer, and women with diets high in beta-carotene and vitamin E have less risk of developing breast cancer. So powerful is the effect of beta-carotene that it can actually reverse as well as prevent the abnormal growth of cervical cells, which shows up on Pap smears as a warning signal of cancer.

How does beta-carotene help protect us against cancer? We don't yet know the complete story, but we do know that beta-carotene is a potent stimulator of the immune system. Vitamin A has always been known to stimulate the immune system, but we now know that beta-carotene itself enhances immune function independently of vitamin A. The two, together, pack quite an immune-boosting punch.

Beta-carotene's ability to prevent all forms of cancer is currently being tested by the Harvard Medical School. One of us was asked to participate in the study, but declined. The study is double-blind, meaning that half of the participants will be given carotene and half will be given a placebo. We believe so strongly that carotene is an important nutrient that we don't want to take the chance we'd be given the dummy pills instead of carotene!

B Vitamins—The Extended Family of Nutrition

Have you ever wondered why there are so many B vitamins and only one of all the others? Has it ever occurred to you to ask why there is a B_{12}, but that when you count the actual B vitamins you get only 11?

The answers to these questions are simple. Most of the vitamins were named during the first 20 or 30 years of this century. Scientists were moving into unknown territory, and their equipment and techniques were not as sophisticated as they are today. Originally, they believed that all the nutritional effects of the B vitamins were caused by a single substance, which they called "vitamin B."

Then they started discovering different substances were pulling off the same functions in the body. These were named B_1, B_2, B_3, B_4, B_5, and so on. There was no central research agency in control, so there was little, if any, order to the naming process. Sometimes a scientist would reveal a new function and name a new vitamin to go along with it, only the new vitamin was actually an old vitamin rediscovered in a new function. So endless B vitamins were pulled out of a pool of only a few distinct compounds.

And the term *B complex* is a misnomer also. Though the

B vitamins occur together in foods, share many functions, and overlap in others, they are chemically distinct. If we were naming the vitamins all over again, we probably would want to disband the B complex and give each vitamin its own name. Actually, they already have their own names, and that's how we'll identify them in this book.

Of course, if we were to rename all the vitamins, and include all the essential nutrients that can be cofactors to vital enzyme reactions inside the body, giving them each a letter for a name, we'd need a larger alphabet. We would want to include not only the 16 vitamins, but the essential minerals—and a host of Beyond Vitamins nutrients too.

The B vitamins are water-soluble, which means they are principally active in the water-soluble reactions in the body. The importance of this fact is that B vitamins—and other water-soluble nutrients—are not effectively stored in the body. Most storage occurs in the fatty areas. Because water-soluble vitamins are regularly flushed through and out of the body, sudden deficiencies are easily developed. Any factor that tends to increase the flow of water through the body, such as stress, exertion, and illness do, will also flush water-soluble nutrients out of the body faster.

Thiamine (B_1)—Our Energy Spark

Thiamine is the spark plug of the body's engine. Without adequate thiamine, the burning of sugar for energy falters and a wide range of bodily functions suffers. Acidic waste products of incomplete combustion collect and impair the muscles, brain, nervous system, digestion, heart, lungs, and immune system.

Thiamine supplements have been shown to reduce stuttering among young children, and improve memory. Injections of thiamine and liver extract can give some symptomatic relief from multiple sclerosis.

Riboflavin (B$_2$)—Our Power Regulator

If your car is fuel-injected, it has an electronic circuit that determines the correct air-fuel mixture for maximum energy. Our bodies are also fuel-injected. Our cells need the correct oxygen-blood sugar mixture for efficient operation. Riboflavin is the key cofactor in the biochemical "circuit" that provides that correct mixture. Without enough riboflavin, we run like a car that needs an overhaul. The eyes, nerves, adrenal glands, skin, and mucous membranes deteriorate in a deficiency.

Riboflavin helps us respond to stress. We see better, look better, and behave better when we have enough riboflavin. Our skin and hair need plenty of this vitamin. Our muscles' ability to perform work is supported by riboflavin. Riboflavin also helps detoxify noxious chemicals.

Niacin (B$_3$)—The 3-D Vitamin

Niacin is necessary for the cells to breathe and utilize nutrients. More than 40 different biochemical reactions require adequate niacin. Niacin widens the diameter of the blood vessels and increases blood flow. In many people, high doses cause a temporary reaction known as a "niacin flush"—skin temperature rises, the skin is flushed, blood pressure temporarily drops, and dizziness may occur.

Severe niacin deficiency causes the "3-Ds," or diarrhea, dermatitis, and dementia. This syndrome is known as pellagra. Many years ago, entire hospitals were built just to treat people suffering from pellagra, which was thought to be an infectious disease.

High doses of niacin have been used successfully by physicians in the treatment of mental illness (schizophrenia) and arthritis. Niacin may also help prevent and relieve mild anxiety, apprehension, loss of appetite, fatigue, insomnia, depression, hyperactivity, and other mental disturbances.

Pyridoxine (B₆)—The Key Nutrient

Pyridoxine is a key factor in the body's utilization of protein, carbohydrates, and fats. The cells cannot produce energy, and the body cannot grow, repair, or in any way maintain itself without this vitamin. Pyridoxine supports the nervous system, the bones and teeth—actually, the entire protein and collagen structure of the body. You've seen the toothpaste commercials claiming a reduction in cavities? Well, pyridoxine has reduced cavities by as much as 40 percent in children receiving a 9 mg. supplement.

Pyridoxine also supports the immune system by helping to maintain the thymus gland. Pyridoxine supplements can help alleviate depression and disturbed blood sugar tolerance and carbohydrate metabolism caused by oral contraceptives. Pyridoxine helps relieve premenstrual swelling and acne, and in some women it may help lessen premenstrual tension, depression, and aches and pains. Some physicians have reported that the vitamin relieves arthritis symptoms.

Pyridoxine supplements may also help children with hyperactivity, irritability, autism, and other mental disturbances. Pyridoxine also helps the liver detoxify poisonous chemicals.

Folic Acid—The Anti-Aging Vitamin

Our body's synthesis of DNA and RNA, proteins that are required for cell reproduction, depends on folic acid (also called folate). We've all heard the maxim that the body completely reproduces itself every seven years. Well, however long it takes, the body is constantly replacing old cells. Then why do we age? Some scientists believe it's because the cells' ability to reproduce copies of themselves begins to deteriorate, thus producing fewer and fewer efficient copies. Some scientists believe the cause of this deterioration is a falling off of the quality of our DNA and RNA. In light of this, folic acid may someday be thought of as an anti-aging vitamin.

We may already have enough information to satisfy the requirements for the title. Folic acid supports the immune system, bone marrow, hair, mucous membranes, red blood cells, fingernails, and nervous system. Folic acid has been used to help relieve the symptoms of mental patients and mothers suffering from postpartum depression. Confusion, disorientation, depression, and other symptoms which, when they occur in old people are called "senility," often respond to folic acid treatments. Folic acid also helps support balanced blood sugar levels. Folic acid supplements have helped relieve symptoms of psoriasis, and gingivitis, or gum inflammation, may also respond to these supplements.

Cobalamin (B_{12})—Folic Acid's Partner

Cobalamin appears to work alongside folic acid. The body's utilization of folic acid, DNA and RNA synthesis, and the nervous system all depend on cobalamin. Classic cobalamin deficiency is called pernicious anemia, which produces deterioration of the nervous system, which can be fatal. Until the cure for pernicious anemia was discovered in 1926, the disease killed more than 6,000 people every year in the United States alone.

Cobalamin supports the immune system and the nervous system. The vitamin has been used successfully in the treatment of mental illness. Often, the vitamin is injected rather than taken orally. Many persons are unable to absorb cobalamin because of a lack of the necessary digestive factor. Thousands of middle-aged and elderly people do not let a week go by without their cobalamin injections, which they claim gives them more energy and helps them feel better.

Biotin—For Youthful Skin

Biotin is required for the synthesis of protein and fatty acids and the utilization of carbohydrates. It supports the thyroid and adrenal glands, the reproductive organs, the nervous system, immune system, and the skin.

Pantothenic Acid—The Stress Vitamin

Every cell in the body depends on a constant supply of pantothenate. But our adrenal glands appear to need more than any other organ. Stress taxes the adrenals and uses up pantothenate. The immune system is also supported by this vitamin.

Pantothenate strengthens our response to stress and speeds healing, and it helps protect us against radiation and allergens. Animal experiments have demonstrated that pantothenate prolongs life.

Choline—The Brain Booster

Choline exists in the body in such large amounts, particularly in the brain and nervous system, that it may be more a macronutrient or a structural component than a micronutrient or catalyst. Choline also helps protect the liver against toxic chemicals.

Choline has been used effectively to treat several disorders of the nervous system, including tardive dyskinesia, Huntington's chorea, Gille de la Tourette's syndrome, Friedrich's ataxia, manic depression, and Alzheimer's disease. Choline supplements can also help improve memory and mental efficiency in healthy people.

Inositol—For Your Nerves

Inositol supports and protects the nervous system, and has been used to prevent the degeneration of nerve insulation that sometimes occurs in diabetes. This vitamin also helps the liver detoxify poisons.

PABA—Keeps Your Skin Light and Your Hair Dark

PABA, or paraaminobenzoic acid, is known as the anti-gray hair vitamin. In animal experiments, a deficiency of PABA results in gray hair. Although controlled experiments do not exist that show PABA's effectiveness in restoring color to human gray hair, there are several clinical and personal reports that high doses are effective.

PABA, applied directly to the skin, is an effective sunscreen, and most protective sun lotions contain varying amounts of PABA.

Vitamin C—A Mountain of Benefits

When it comes to writing about vitamin C, an author has no problem digging up evidence of the vitamin's usefulness to maintaining good health. Rather, the problem is sorting through mountains of evidence!

To get an idea just how important vitamin C really is, imagine what would happen to your house if all the nails, glue, and cement were removed. The house would fall apart, of course. But imagine how bad the devastation would be if not only the nails, glue, and cement were removed, but the microscopic glue that holds the molecules of wood, mortar, and other materials was also removed. You'd be left with a pile of dust.

Vitamin C is essential to the formation of collagen, which is the fundamental glue of the body. Collagen is a protein that supports bone, skin, teeth, muscle, cartilage, tendon, and connective tissue. Without adequate vitamin C, the body begins literally to disintegrate into dust. Stress uses up vitamin C. Conversely, vitamin C supports our ability to withstand stress. The vitamin also helps the cells breathe, and serves as a powerful antioxidant.

Vitamin C boosts the immune system, encourages healing, and supports fertility. The vitamin helps us better withstand stress of all kinds, including temperature stress. The strength of the blood vessels depends on vitamin C. Vitamin C supplements raise HDL cholesterol (the good kind, because it's on its way out of the body) and lower LDL cholesterol (the bad kind, because it's on its way into the cells).

In Linus Pauling's research, vitamin C has shown promise in prolonging the lives of terminal cancer patients. In some cases, it can lower insulin requirements for diabetics. The vitamin detoxifies many common pollutants and poisons.

Vitamin D—The Sunshine Vitamin We Can Make Ourselves

Vitamin D is actually a hormone that encourages the absorption of calcium and phosphorus from the intestine and controls the deposit of these minerals in the bones and teeth. Adequate vitamin D supplementation helps prevent osteoporosis.

Vitamin D is called the sunshine vitamin because the body can make its own when we're exposed to sufficient sunlight. In the northern fall and winter, however, the oblique angle of solar radiation makes it almost impossible to get enough vitamin D by natural synthesis. Also, healthy liver and kidneys are needed to make vitamin D. The elderly, or people with kidney damage, may not be able to synthesize enough. Nevertheless, high-dose supplementation of vitamin D is not a good idea, because high doses can suppress the immune system. We recommend no more than baseline supplementation. Also, be aware that fortified dairy products contain artificial vitamin D_2, which is potentially more toxic than the natural form.

Vitamin E—Our Protector

Vitamin E's major role is as an antioxidant that protects the fatty acids in and around the cells from free radical chemical damage. Because free radical oxidation has been implicated in such a wide range of problems—from aging to immune deficiency—vitamin E is a very important nutrient. Vitamin E protects and supports the sex glands and sexual function, the immune system, the endocrine glands, the blood, and the nerves. The vitamin helps determine how well we respond to and withstand stress, through its support of the endocrine system and its role in protecting against free radical damage. One of the ways stress harms is through the creation of extra free radicals.

Vitamin E can encourage healing when applied directly to viral sores and other minor wounds. Vitamin E also decreases the blood's tendency to clot, which is of some value to people with cardiovascular disease.

Vitamin E helps protect us against air pollution, particularly ozone, and also against the free radical damage caused by radiation.

VITAMIN E—THE SEX VITAMIN AFTER ALL?

Remember a few years back when vitamin E first became one of the vitamin superstars? It was proclaimed "the sex vitamin," because the early work establishing it as an essential nutrient revealed that it was essential to fertility. Although headline writers kept calling it the sex vitamin, those who wrote the articles took great pains to explain that vitamin E did not enhance sexual performance.

Well, we may have jumped the gun on disclaiming the vitamin's role in strengthening sexual desire. In our chapter on sex (Chapter 9) we explain why vitamin E may be the sex vitamin after all, especially for women.

Whether you care if it's the sex vitamin or not, vitamin E is a vital part of the Beyond Vitamins program for many other reasons. New studies confirm that vitamin E can help make breast cysts disappear. The vitamin may do this by increasing production of adrenal hormones, thus helping the body maintain hormonal balance.

New research reveals that vitamin E apparently has some anti-inflammatory effect too, since it has been found to reduce the pain suffered in osteoarthritis. The vitamin can also help reduce gum inflammation and tartar.

New research has also found that in combination with the mineral selenium, vitamin E is a potent immune stimulant. Together with vitamin C, vitamin E can detoxify mutagenic, cancer-causing materials in the bowel.

MINERALS

Calcium—For Strong Bones and Steady Nerves

Some minerals have roles similar to the vitamins, as cofactors in biochemical reactions. Some are used as structural components of the body. A few minerals, such as calcium, have both roles. The body contains over 3 pounds of calcium, 99 percent of which is in the bones and teeth. The remaining 1 percent is responsible for the strength of the membranes between the cells and also is a cofactor in many enzyme reactions. Calcium in part regulates the irritability of the nerves and muscles. When calcium is low, the muscles and nerves become more tense and excitable.

The calcium in the bones and teeth is not deposited for life. If blood levels of the mineral fall too low, calcium is drawn out of the bones and teeth to maintain adequate blood levels. Adequate dietary levels of calcium are required to maintain the strength of the bones. Otherwise, they become progressively more porous and weak as we get older. In women, this process appears to begin as early as the midtwenties. In men it begins about a decade later.

Calcium supplements can not only prevent osteoporosis, or loss of bone density and strength, but they can reverse it as well. Although the news media have been trumpeting this fact as if it had just been discovered, there's been abundant evidence available for more than a decade.

Calcium supplements tend to lower blood levels of cholesterol and tryglycerides, by binding with these fats in the digestive tract. We also know that adequate calcium is required for maintaining normal blood pressure. People with diets higher in calcium tend to have lower blood pressure. Calcium also apparently plays a role in preventing cancer, by detoxifying potentially cancer-causing compounds in the bowel.

Chromium—The Energy Factor

Five to ten years from now the news media will be making a fuss about chromium, but you can get the same information now.

We all need chromium, and evidence suggests that many of us aren't getting nearly enough of this vital mineral. Two factors cause chromium loss: stress and sugar in the diet. Taking into consideration the 100 or so pounds of sugar most of us consume every year, plus the fact that chromium is removed when whole foods are processed, it should come as no surprise that the USDA itself found that most Americans are deficient in chromium.

Chromium plays a vital role in the body's utilization of blood sugar, as a cofactor in the hormone insulin's regulation of sugar uptake by the cells. The mineral, in the form in which it is active as a cofactor in blood sugar uptake—glucose tolerance factor—has been shown to eliminate or reduce the insulin requirements of diabetics and also to increase the energy efficiency of healthy people. Chromium's normalizing effect on the body's energy supply was discovered in 1853. Liver and brewer's yeast are very high in GTF-chromium, and most supplements are derived from those foods.

Chromium also plays a role in the prevention of cardiovascular disease. Chromium supplements appear to lower blood levels of cholesterol and reduce the incidence of atherosclerotic plaques.

Copper—The Controversial Mineral

Copper is required to maintain proper pigmentation of skin and hair, the elastic quality of blood vessels, the structural integrity of the bones and nerves, and our sense of taste. Copper supplementation is controversial in that some people argue that we don't get enough (because of zinc supplementation) and some that we get too much (because of copper water pipes and other reasons). We believe that there is no reason at this time to take special supplements of copper, except in trace amounts as part of a multimineral supplement.

Iodine—One of the First Supplements

Iodine is required for the synthesis of thyroxin, or thyroid hormone, which regulates the body's metabolic rate. Iodine is also used by the white blood cells to destroy bacteria and other disease-causing organisms. Iodine deficiency disease, goiter, still affects more than 200 million people around the world. In the United States, iodine deficiency is extremely rare. Even people with goiter appear to have a problem absorbing or utilizing their iodine, rather than getting enough in the diet. There does not appear to be any evidence recommending special supplements other than what occurs in iodized salt and multimineral supplements.

Iron—Please Use Discretion

Iron supports the blood's ability to carry oxygen to the cells. If there's not enough iron, the cells don't "breathe" as well as they need to in order to provide energy. Iron supplementation is most important for women and for children of both sexes. Men usually do not need special iron supplements, apart from what's contained in multimineral supplements.

The body purposely lowers blood levels of iron during infections, and there is some evidence that high blood levels of iron can encourage bacterial infections. Of course, a serious iron deficiency can be even more detrimental to the immune system. Still, the risks of oversupplementation are real. There is new evidence that excess iron generates very potent and damaging free radicals.

We advise discretion in the use of iron supplements. Only pregnant, lactating, and menstruating women and persons who have lost, or continue to lose blood require iron supplementation. When selecting a multivitamin-mineral supplement, look for one that contains little or no iron.

Magnesium—The Master Mineral

Magnesium not only plays a role in many enzyme reactions, but it also happens to be *the* central element in the control of cell metabolism and growth. Magnesium is the master mineral of the cell and, thus, of the body.

Magnesium supports healthy levels of nerve and muscle excitability, and prevents tremors, spasms, convulsions, and cramps. Magnesium helps keep us wide awake, full of energy, alert, strong, and balanced. Not only is fatigue a symptom of magnesium deficiency, but psychosis and mental disturbances as well.

Recent research reveals that magnesium has a role in preventing heart disease, relieving angina pains, lowering high blood pressure, and preventing toxemia of pregnancy. Intravenous infusions of magnesium given immediately after a heart attack can prevent the spread of damage.

Manganese—For Balanced Blood Sugar

Manganese plays important roles in the synthesis of DNA and RNA, protein, cartilage, and the body's use of insulin to regulate blood sugar. African folk medicine uses alfalfa, which is high in manganese, in the treatment of diabetes. Contemporary doctors have also made use of manganese to treat and prevent disturbances in blood sugar balance. The mineral has also been used to relieve seizures caused by convulsive disorders in children and side effects of psychiatric drugs.

Molybdenum—Rare but Essential

Some minerals, such as manganese, exist almost everywhere. Some, like molybdenum, are quite rare. Nevertheless, molybdenum is an essential nutrient. It acts as a cofactor in several enzyme systems—particularly energy production. There is no evidence to suggest that it is necessary to take special supplements of molybdenum other than what might be contained in a multimineral. Molybdenum seems to play a supportive role in iron absorption.

Phosphorus—Essential, but Rarely Needed

Phosphorus may very well be the single most essential mineral, judging from its requirement for more biochemical functions than any other mineral. There is no need to take supplements of phosphorus, however, because our food supply is more likely to contain too much rather than not enough.

Potassium—For Your Heart's Strength

To get an idea of how important potassium is, consider the fact that an adult carries more than a half pound of the mineral in his or her body at all times—all of it in the soft tissues or fluids of the body. Potassium is involved in the excitability of nerves and the contraction of muscles. In addition to many enzyme reactions within the cells, potassium supports the rhythmic beating of the heart and the strength of the muscles. Potassium helps counteract the blood pressure-raising effects of sodium. A recent study found that people with higher potassium intakes have a significantly lower incidence of strokes.

Selenium—Trace Mineral with a Mountain of Benefits

Selenium is a potent antioxidant and immune system stimulant. Several vital enzyme systems, the muscles, hair, skin, nails, the red blood cells, DNA-RNA synthesis, cellular respiration and energy transfer, production of sperm, and glucose tolerance depend on it. Selenium also plays a role in preventing heart disease and cancer.

Silicon—Our Ubiquitous Friend

Silicon, which is the most abundant mineral on earth, also happens to be an essential nutrient. The concentration of silicon in our blood is the same as in sea water. The parts of the body that contain higher proportions, and that are particularly dependent on an adequate supply, are the brain, heart, muscles, hair, ligaments, liver, lungs, bones, and blood vessels. Silicon shows great promise as a promoter of healing and calcification of the bones. It also has a role in retarding the aging process and preventing heart disease.

Zinc—The Super Mineral

Without adequate zinc, the cells could not breathe, grow, or reproduce. Zinc is a good antioxidant and a powerful immune stimulant. In many malnourished people, zinc supplements alone are often enough to restore immune competence. It's required to protect us against stress and infections, and to promote speedy healing. Zinc supplements can cut in half the amount of time required to heal after surgery.

Zinc plays a very important role in male sexual potency. The prostate gland requires a constant, adequate supply of zinc, and semen contains high amounts of the mineral. Zinc supplements have helped reduce the inflammation of chronic, noninfectious prostatitis. Zinc also plays a role in the production of the male hormone, testosterone. Zinc supplements have been used successfully to restore potency to men with low testosterone and zinc levels.

Zinc supplements have also been shown to be beneficial in treating acne and rheumatoid arthritis. We believe zinc to be an important anti-inflammatory nutrient. It stabilizes the lysosomal membranes within the cell. The lysosomes contain enzymes and free radicals which, if the membranes are ruptured, can cause the cells to self-destruct, thus causing inflammation.

AMINO ACIDS

We now know that many of the amino acids not only serve as structural components of proteins, but also serve as factors in various crucial biochemical functions, just as the vitamins and minerals do. And, beyond vitamin- and mineral-type functions, the amino acids are also critical to the function of the brain.

We also know that though several amino acids can be made by the body, it doesn't necessarily mean that the body is making enough for all of its needs. Evidence suggests that various factors may prevent the body from synthesizing enough amino acids. In some cases the diet does not supply enough raw materials. In others, diseases or stresses of all kinds combine with genetic and metabolic factors to cause amino acid deficiencies. In years to come, amino acids may equal vitamins and minerals as therapeutic agents in sickness, and preventive agents in health.

Now we're going to introduce the amino acids.

Aspartic Acid—A Good Partner for Minerals

Aspartic acid may help lessen fatigue and boost endurance. Teamed up with potassium, calcium, and magnesium it supports the cardiovascular system. As a detoxifier, it protects the nervous system against excess ammonia by helping to remove the chemical from the body.

Aspartic acid is a good mineral chelator, or binder. Used in supplements of calcium, magnesium, zinc, and potassium-magnesium (as mineral-aspartates), it increases absorption and utilization of the minerals.

Carnitine Helps the Body Burn Fat

Carnitine is required for the body to burn fatty acids for fuel, and is vital to fat metabolism, especially in the heart and skeletal muscles. By stimulating the efficiency with which the cells burn fat, carnitine helps lower blood levels of triglycerides and other blood fats.

Although carnitine can be manufactured by the body, in many people this is not sufficient. Adequate quantities of the amino acids lysine and methionine are required for carnitine synthesis. Although high-quality protein contains plenty of lysine and methionine, unbalanced vegetarian diets may be deficient, thus causing a carnitine deficiency. Carnitine deficiencies may also stem from enzyme deficiencies. A deficiency can cause fatty liver, high blood fats, muscle wasting and weakness, weakened immune system, loss of sex drive, infertility, and heart failure.

Carnitine may be of use to dieters. Weight-loss diets usually produce high blood levels of toxic by-products of fat metabolism, called ketones. Ketosis can be fatal if these ketones build up to a high enough concentration. Carnitine, however, can minimize the buildup of ketones, by accelerating fat metabolism.

Cysteine Is a Major Detoxifier

Cysteine is vital to the formation of keratin, the dominant protein in hair, skin, and nails. It can also work as an antioxidant, together with vitamin E and selenium, to protect the body from free radicals. Cysteine is also an effective chelator of toxic heavy metals. It binds with lead, mercury, and cadmium, forms an insoluble complex, and pulls them out of the body. Garlic is very high in cysteine.

Cystine—All Around Booster

Cystine is vital to the immune system because it is used in the formation of antibodies. The blood-sugar regulating hormone insulin also requires cystine for its manufacture. Cystine also supports rapid healing from wounds, surgery, and burns. As a detoxifier, it helps protect the body from alcohol and environmental pollution.

Glutamine for Your Sweet Tooth

Glutamine works to reduce our craving for sweets and alcohol. It also improves memory and mental acuity and helps stave off fatigue and depression. The body generally makes its own glutamine, and blood levels are usually the highest of any amino acid. These levels tend to be low in people with hypoglycemia, however. During starvation, the brain can directly metabolize glutamine.

Glycine—The First Amino Acid

Glycine is the biochemically simplest amino acid, and was probably the first made by nature. Glycine supports the prostate gland, the muscles, and the nervous system. It slow down nerve transmissions, decreases seizures and may slow down heart arrythmias. Sweet to the taste, this amino acid is a natural antacid.

Histidine Promises Relief for Allergies

Histidine increases circulation by widening the blood vessels, and has been used in the treatment of anemia. It can also help lessen or prevent allergic reactions. (*Caution:* See Chapter 10 before using histidine in an attempt to reduce allergic reactions. It should be done only under supervision, because it may intensify, rather than reduce, the reaction in some people.)

Isoleucine—A Link in the Energy Chain

Isoleucine helps balance blood sugar. It is combined with leucine and valine to treat certain enzyme defects. Isoleucine, leucine, and valine are classed as branched-chain amino acids. The muscle cells seem to prefer these amino acids and use them for energy production before they use others. Branched-chain amino acids may help boost stamina and muscular endurance. They are also used to prevent low blood sugar.

Leucine—Another Energy Link

Leucine plays a role in the regulation of blood sugar and also supports the healing of trauma to skin and bones. In some persons, however, leucine supplements can cause low blood sugar.

Lysine—The Antiviral Amino Acid

Lysine strengthens the immune system, stimulates tissue repair, supports the manufacture of hormones and enzymes, and promotes bone development through its stimulation of calcium absorption. It is also used by the body to make carnitine. Lysine supplements have proved useful in the treatment of herpes virus infections.

Methionine Is a Potent Detoxifier

The body needs a daily supply of sulphur, and methionine is our primary amino acid source. Methionine supports the liver and the digestive system, and promotes the healthy metabolism of fats. It is known as a "lipotrope" because it helps reduce a fatty liver, which is present in persons who consume high levels of alcohol and/or sugar.

Ornithine—The Youth Extender

Ornithine stimulates the immune system and the healing process. Along with arginine, it plays an important role in fat metabolism and the release of growth hormone.

L-Phenylalanine—The "Up" Amino Acid

The "L" form of phenylalanine boosts the formation of noradrenaline and dopamine, neurotransmitters in the brain that promote normal appetite, increase mental alertness, and stabilize mood swings. Because phenylalanine may constrict the blood vessels, it should not be used by persons with high blood pressure or cardiovascular disease.

DL-Phenylalanine—For Chronic Pain

The "DL" form of phenylalanine, a combination of the "D" and the "L" forms, has a pain-reducing effect. Actually, it is the "D" form that reduces pain, by boosting levels of endorphins, the body's own pain relievers. It is less expensive to manufacture the "DL" form, however. Headaches and chronic back pain seem to be the most responsive to this amino acid. It also can help relieve depression.

Taurine—The Natural Tranquilizer

Together with glycine, taurine supports balance in the nervous system by slowing down nerve impulses. In this way it acts as a tranquilizer, alleviating insomnia, anxiety, hyperactivity, and seizures. It may also be useful in lowering heart arrythmias.

Threonine Keeps Skin Youthful

Threonine plays a role in the formation of collagen, elastin, and the enamel protein of nails and teeth. It supports healthy fat metabolism and liver function.

Tryptophan—Antidepressant and Sleep Aid

Tryptophan is an important amino acid for balancing brain activity through its effect on levels of the brain neurotransmitter serotonin, which induces sleep and stimulates dreaming. Tryptophan supplements can alleviate insomnia, resulting in sleep that comes sooner and lasts longer. Tryptophan can also act as an antidepressant and a natural tranquilizer, and has been successfully used to relieve the pain of headaches, arthritis, migraine, muscle and backaches, and other chronic conditions. It may be of help in stabilizing appetite swings and withdrawal from nicotine.

Tryptophan is most effective when taken with fruit juice, sweetened milk, and pyridoxine (B_6).

Tyrosine—The Mood Booster

Tyrosine plays a role in the production of melanin, the pigment that lends color to hair and skin. The thyroid gland uses tyrosine and iodine to manufacture thyroid hormone. Tyrosine also boosts mental alertness and aids in the treatment of allergies and headaches.

Tyrosine raises brain levels of noradrenaline and dopamine, as does phenylalanine. (Phenylalanine is actually converted to tyrosine in the body.) There have been partially successful efforts to treat Parkinson's disease, in which dopamine levels are low, by administering tyrosine and (phosphatidyl) choline.

Valine—Third Link in the Energy Chain

Valine is useful in restoring healthy amino acid balance, which has been damaged by addictions to drugs, chemicals, or certain foods. Together with leucine and isoleucine, valine supports muscle function.

Peptides—The Cutting Edge of Amino Acid Research

Peptides are small compounds consisting of from 2 to 10 amino acids. We have discovered just recently that peptides play very important roles as hormones and neurotransmitters. For example, it's been known for a relatively long time that the posterior pituitary hormones regulate uterine contractions and water retention, and that alcohol causes urination by inhibiting the peptide responsible for water retention.

Lately, new roles have been discovered for peptides. They also appear to stimulate the immune system and boost the production of interferon (an important immune warrior) and endorphins (the body's "feel good" chemicals). Through genetic recombination technology, we are now able to mass-produce peptides.

ENZYMES

If we don't have enough digestive enzymes, food particles will not be broken down small enough for adequate absorption to take place. Some of the nutrients from our food and our supplements can be wasted, and this becomes a critical problem as we get older. After the age of 40, levels of hydrochloric acid and digestive enzymes begin to decrease. As we get older, we're more likely to become victims of poor absorption and multiple nutritional deficiencies, even though we may be eating a diet that was adequate for us when we were younger.

Inadequate supplies of digestive enzymes may also allow many undigested, or partially digested, larger-than-normal protein molecules to be passed along to the intestines. Many of these incomplete breakdown products wind up in the bloodstream and cause allergic reactions.

Pancreatic Enzymes for Digestion

If you're not digesting your food completely, you probably do not have enough pancreatic enzymes. The pancreas secretes protein-, starch-, and fat-digesting enzymes into the small intestine in response to the acidity of the stomach contents. So if your stomach is deficient in hydrochloric acid, the food entering the intestines will not be sufficiently acidic, and your pancreas will not secrete enough enzymes to digest your food properly. Usually, digestive enzyme supplementation includes betaine hydrochloride or glutamic acid hydrochloride to increase stomach acidity and pancreatic enzymes or pancreatin to improve digestion.

Many factors can interfere with proper, complete digestion. If you're under stress or upset before a meal, hydrochloric acid and enzyme secretion may be diminished. If a meal does not contain enough amino acids, especially tryptophan and/or phenylalanine, enzyme secretion may be lessened. Illness or chronic malnutrition will also decrease our ability to produce enzymes. Overconsumption of specific foods will lessen the supply of enzymes needed to digest those foods. The pancreas adapts to our habitual diet, so if we switch diets quickly, before the gland can adapt its patterns of enzyme secretion, incomplete digestion can result.

Anti-Inflammatory Enzymes

Proteolytic enzymes (in combination with vitamin C and bioflavonoids) can be more effective than aspirin for reducing pain, swelling, edema, and heat of inflammation caused by injury. Trypsin, chymotrypsin, papain (from papaya),

bromelain (from pineapple), and streptokinase (from strep-
tococcus bacteria) can be used to reduce soreness and speed
the healing of bruises resulting from mild athletic injuries.
Papain and bromelain have been used successfully to reduce pain and swelling after oral surgery.

This ability of proteolytic enzymes to digest protein may
someday be of use in helping us fight off viral infections.
Viruses cannot take hold unless their protein coating is
intact. Proteolytic enzymes have demonstrated the ability
to digest that coating and destroy the viruses.

GLANDULAR SUPPLEMENTS

Glandular therapy is one of the oldest forms of medicine
and glandular concentrates were among the very first supplements.

Glandular therapy is relatively simple. If you know what
organ or gland is ailing, or what gland controls the specific
function you want to heal, you need only to find a supplement that contains the concentrate from that organ or
gland.

In the remaining pages of this section, we will describe
some glandular supplements and briefly explain their potential value.

Heart tissue, for example, has been shown to stimulate
the regeneration of the heart muscle in controlled animal
experiments.

Testicular concentrate may stimulate regeneration of
the testes and improve sexual functioning.

Raw liver concentrate was actually one of the first supplements. In Ershoff's classic animal experiments, liver
concentrate boosted strength, endurance, performance, and
resistance to stress and disease. The effect was not due to
the vitamins and minerals in the liver. The control group

of animals that did not receive liver was given supplements of all the known vitamins and minerals in liver. Still, their performance did not come close to that of the liver-supplemented animals.

Liver tissue not only supports and restores the healthy function of the liver, but also helps balance the blood sugar. There is no mystery about how liver improves the body's utilization of blood sugar—liver is an excellent source of glucose tolerance factor, the form of chromium that is required for sugar metabolism. Liver concentrate also helps reduce fatty deposits in the liver, and also contains substances that stimulate regeneration of the liver.

The pancreas has two major functions. One is to secrete insulin, the hormone that regulates the cells' uptake of blood sugar. The other is to secrete digestive enzymes. Pancreas concentrate does help balance the blood sugar. In fact, before insulin was used, pancreas concentrate was the treatment of choice for diabetes.

Pancreatic concentrate also supplies digestive enzymes that can boost digestive efficiency, enhance absorption of nutrients, relieve inflammation, reduce bacterial overgrowth in the gastrointestinal tract, and restore healthful intestinal flora.

Pancreas concentrate also provides picolinic acid, a substance that enhances zinc absorption and availability to the tissues by a factor of 500 percent. Picolinic acid is also found in human milk.

Duodenum concentrate helps support the duodenal mucosa, which is vital to the absorption of nutrients. Duodenum also heals and protects the digestive tract from ulcers, and together with stomach concentrate and pancreatic enzymes, enhances the absorption of vitamin B_{12}.

Stomach concentrate not only increases B_{12} absorption by providing "intrinsic factor," the enzyme that promotes B_{12} absorption, but also helps prevent and repair ulcerative damage to the stomach and duodenum. Stomach concentrate contains high levels of pepsin, an enzyme that works with hydrochloric acid to release B_{12} and other nutrients from food.

Bone marrow concentrate was used with success to restore immune capacity and red blood cell production long before the modern bone marrow transplants—as far back as 1896. Modern use of bone marrow concentrate might include boosting the immune system and protecting the body from radiation damage.

The thymus gland is a major controlling gland of the immune system. It is a "teacher" gland that instructs vital soldiers in our immune "army" how to select and destroy enemy organisms and foreign invaders. The thymus gland, however, shrinks as we grow older. Properly prepared thymus concentrate contains thymosin, the thymus hormone that stimulates and "teaches" the immune system.

Thymus extract has been used successfully to boost immune power in persons with weakened immunity. It was found that the thymosin did not have to survive the GI tract in order to be effective. Fragments of the thymus protein, or peptides, entering the bloodstream were sufficient to stimulate immune competency.

The spleen is the largest lymphoid organ in the body, and it cooperates with the thymus as a part of the immune system. White blood cells and other cells that consume and destroy invading cells and molecules are formed and stored in the spleen. When needed, these white blood cells, or lymphocytes, are discharged en masse. We know that vigorous exercise can double the amount of lymphocytes in the blood. New red blood cells are also stored in the spleen, and old ones are filtered out of the bloodstream.

Spleen concentrate and extract has been used since 1929 for support and stimulation of the immune system, and specifically in the treatment of people with Hodgkin's disease. Injected spleen extract has an antiviral action similar to interferon and is capable of detoxifying bacterial toxins.

Spleen concentrate may contain thymus-stimulating factors, and may not only heal spleen and bone marrow, but also enhance resistance to abnormal cell growth.

Spleen concentrate also has been shown to help protect animals from radiation damage, not only by speeding the recovery of the spleen and bone marrow, but in a general nutritional way by protecting the skin. In other animal experiments, spleen extract also enhanced the regeneration of the thymus gland after radiation exposure. Spleen concentrate has anti-inflammatory and antiblood clotting properties, and it enhances lymphatic function in the entire body.

The adrenal glands govern our response to stress, infections, physical and mental challenges, allergens, and sexual stimulation. Adrenal concentrate may be useful in supporting all of these activities. Adrenal extract is known to contain active enzymes, which help the body transform cholesterol into adrenal hormones.

A combination of hypothalamus, pituitary, and adrenal concentrates may normalize endocrine balance and relieve certain forms of depression, anxiety, insomnia, and fatigue. Many vitamins must be converted to their active forms before they can be used by the body, a process that relies on stimulation by the adrenal glands and the pituitary gland. Concentrates of these glands may then enhance absorption of nutrients.

The *thyroid gland* regulate the body's entire metabolism. A person with an underactive thyroid gland may become tired, anemic, prone to infections, and have difficulty keeping warm; he or she may find it hard to lose weight, and may lose interest in sex. Thyroid concentrate may help to alleviate these problems, although most people with chronically underactive thyroid glands require supplementation with actual thyroid hormone.

Bone concentrate or bone meal is, again, a very time-honored supplement. Bone meal is an excellent source of calcium.

Lung concentrate is used for support of the lungs during coughs, colds, respiratory infections, and smoking. It can also be used to improve reduced functional capacity of the lungs.

OTHER BEYOND VITAMINS SUPPLEMENTS

Bioflavonoids

Bioflavonoids are not vitamins. When an essential vitamin or mineral is removed from the diet, specific deficiency symptoms eventually occur. This doesn't happen when bioflavonoids are experimentally removed from the diet. Bioflavonoids truly come into their own as supplements, as nutrients that are added to the diet to boost or regulate biological functions in a healthful way.

Bioflavonoids exist only in plants. Most of the yellow, red, and blue pigmentation in plants comes from the bioflavonoids. The principal sources of bioflavonoids are citrus fruits, particularly lemons and sweet oranges, but they are also derived from buckwheat and other plants. Though there are over 800 naturally-occurring flavonoids, the three commonly used in supplements are rutin, quercetin, and hesperidin.

Bioflavonoids exert their effects in three ways: through the strengthening of membrane and small blood vessel walls, by serving as antioxidants, and by regulating various enzymes. The cement substance that holds the walls of the membranes and blood vessels together is thickened by flavonoids, and they become less fragile and less likely to leak. In this way, when there is an injury, inflammation is reduced because the amount of tissue damage and leaking of blood and fluids into the area is minimized. Bioflavonoids also reduce inflammation by deactivating enzymes that produce inflammation, and by preventing the mast cells from discharging histamine and other inflammatory substances.

Bioflavonoids may be of help in cardiovascular disease not only because they strengthen the blood vessels and reduce inflammation, but also because they decrease the tendency of red blood cells to stick together, forming potentially dangerous clots.

The capillary-strengthening, anti-inflammatory effects of bioflavonoids also account for their use in reducing allergies. Food allergies can result when larger-than-normal, incompletely broken down particles of protein leak through the intestinal wall into the bloodstream. Bioflavonoids help prevent such leaking by optimizing the efficiency of the barrier to the bloodstream. And, of course, their enzyme-deactivating anti-inflammatory effect also helps decrease the effects of allergens that do get through.

Bioflavonoids speed healing in ulcers, periodontal disease, bleeding disorders, and injuries by strengthening the tiny blood vessels that tend to rupture, and by reducing inflammation, which sometimes slows healing.

Bioflavonoids have demonstrated effectiveness in boosting the body's protection against viruses, bacteria, and fungi. They apparently boost the immune system in more than one way. By reducing inflammation and allergic responses, they leave the immune system stronger to fight infections. Bioflavonoids are known to deactivate enzymes that produce symptoms in viral infections. And flavonoids also boost the effectiveness of vitamin C, most likely by preserving the vitamin from oxidation and conversion in the body and thus making it more available to the tissues. Studies have shown that a bioflavonoid and vitamin C combination can cut the healing time of herpes sores on the lips by almost two-thirds.

Bioflavonoids may one day be the treatment of choice to prevent cataracts, because they can deactivate the enzyme, aldose reductase, which causes some types of cataracts, particularly those most common in diabetics. The enzyme converts blood sugar, which is often abnormally high in diabetics, into sorbitol, which accumulates and crystalizes in the lens of the eye. Not only do the sorbitol crystals affect the transmission of light through the lens, but they also soak up water and cause increased pressure and tissue damage. In animal experiments, bioflavonoid supplements inhibit the development of diabetic cataracts.

Bioflavonoids not only deactivate potentially harmful enzymes, they also stimulate helpful ones. They are known to boost activity of certain enzymes that inactivate and convert toxic, carcinogenic pollutants into forms that can be excreted from the body.

Essential Oils

Certain essential oils are better for us than others, and some oils are not only essential in the same way that vitamins and minerals are, but some oils can also have quite remarkable effects on health when they are included in the diet.

The essential fatty acids (EFAs) have the same importance to the body as vitamins, in that they are required for certain metabolic reactions to take place, and because the body cannot manufacture them. In fact, they were originally identified as vitamin F. When the diet is deficient in the EFAs, certain predictable symptoms develop, including hair loss, dry skin, painful joints, decline in liver function, fatigue, nervousness, sexual and fertility problems, and increased susceptibility to infections.

Essential fatty acids also regulate the production of hormonelike substances called prostaglandins. There are several forms of prostaglandins, and the body requires a certain balance in order to remain healthy. Recent research has revealed, however, that in many people the biochemical steps that produce prostaglandin 1, PG1, from linoleic acid are somehow blocked. Whether because of genetic or dietary factors, many people are lacking in one very important step: the conversion of linoleic acid to gamma-linolenic acid, or GLA. The enzyme responsible for the conversion is there, but may be diminished in activity because of aging, a high-saturated fat diet, or deficiencies of B₆, magnesium, or zinc. Fortunately, GLA is available in certain oils, including that of the evening primrose plant and the black currant seed.

GLA supplements have been used to relieve premenstrual syndrome, slightly improve the condition of people with multiple sclerosis, lower blood levels of cholesterol, reduce the tendency of the blood to clot, improve circulation and relieve pain in people with intermittent claudication, restore healthy skin condition in people with eczema, relieve inflammation and pain in arthritis, reduce the toxic effects of alcohol, improve resistance to cancer, and strengthen the immune system.

Other important essential fatty acids have been discovered to have great anti-inflammatory, preventive properties. These oils, EPA (eicosapentaenoic acid) and DHA (docosahexaenoic acid) are most commonly present in the oils of cold-water fish, such as cod, mackerel, sardines, herring, kippers, tuna, bonita, pilchard, butterfish, bluefish, and salmon. However, they are also found in the oils of Arctic animals such as polar bears and seals. All wild animals have some of these oils, but the concentrations fall off dramatically in domestic livestock.

EPA and DHA also stimulate the production of anti-inflammatory prostaglandins. They lower blood levels of LDL cholesterol, which is the harmful kind, and increase levels of HDL cholesterol, the helpful kind that is on its way out of the body. EPA and DHA also lower blood levels of other harmful fats, and reduce the tendency of the blood cells to clump together in dangerous clots. They serve to widen the blood vessels, thus reducing the possibility of a heart attack or stroke.

Mucopolysaccharides

Mucopolysaccharides are natural substances that, together with collagen, form the glue that holds together all body tissues. They are responsible not only for the strength of tissues, but also for the transfer of nutrients and other substances through the cell walls.

The mucopolysaccharides can reduce inflammation, speed healing, strengthen the tissues, and stimulate the immune system. They have been used clinically to improve symptoms in arthritis, bursitis, respiratory disease, headaches, ulcers, bedwetting, angina, and allergies. Mucopolysaccharides may also be useful in preventing and reducing the damage done by heart disease.

Finally, these difficult-to-pronounce and even-more-difficult-to-spell nutrients may explain why several foods have gone down in history as aphrodisiacs. Among their many abilities, mucopolysaccharides can boost the production of seminal fluid, and thus stimulate libido and potency. Mussels and oysters, the legendary aphrodisiac sea creatures, contain very high concentration of mucopolysaccharides. So do many other foods that folklore and folk medicine have heralded as aphrodisiacs.

APPENDIX B
Why We Need To Take Supplements

There are still people who believe that supplements don't help us stay healthier. Well, there are also people who believe the earth is flat. That's their right. Unfortunately, many of them would like to force us to believe the same way. They would like to make it against the law to select our own nutritional supplements.

DISCOVER A BOLD
NEW WORLD OF HEALTH

We're convinced that nutritional supplements help us to be healthier and happier. We also believe that it's a good idea to have a solid foundation of confidence that you're doing the right thing for yourself. That's why we're going to spend some time debunking the myth that supplements aren't beneficial.

THANK GOODNESS FOR PACESETTERS

Let's get some perspective on the controversy. The standard medical view is to acknowledge only overt, "classical" signs of nutritional deficiencies. The major problem with this view is the severely limited idea of what "classical signs of nutritional deficiencies" actually are. Unfortunately, the "classical" definitions usually do not include many symptoms that we know from experience as well as from research will respond to nutritional therapy.

For example, at the Cleveland Clinic a large number of people sought medical care, complaining of various symptoms, including craving for sweets (which they all admitted giving in to frequently), abdominal and chest pains, fatigue, sleep disturbances, personality changes, restlessness, and recurrent fever of unknown origin. These people were originally told that there was "nothing wrong with them," and that they should take sedatives and counseling for their anxiety neuroses.

Two physicians at the Cleveland Clinic, however, went a few steps further. First, they tested these people for blood levels of vitamin B_1, or thiamine. The levels were in the "normal" range. Fortunately these doctors knew that blood levels tell only one thing: how much of a given nutrient is in the blood. These numbers are meaningless if a person is still suffering symptoms. Some people need higher blood levels.

The doctors tried something. They gave each of these persons daily supplements of 250 mg of thiamine. Three things happened. Activity of certain vital enzymes known to depend on thiamine shot up. All of their symptoms vanished. And they lost their craving for sweets, which was at the root of the problem in the first place. Sweets drive up our requirements for thiamine.

The point of this example isn't that these symptoms are always caused by a thiamine deficiency. Not at all. Rather, the point is that, unfortunately, we often accept a certain level of impairment of our health, strength, and happiness and call it "normal." Because some government committee has declared that certain amounts of certain nutrients are "adequate," we don't think about what good things might be in store for us if we go beyond these arbitrary definitions of "adequate" and "normal."

We believe we have the right and the ability to explore our own limits of personal health, strength, and fitness—

nutritionally or otherwise. This book is based on the knowledge that providing certain nutrients in amounts that go beyond arbitrary definitions of "normal" and "adequate" can result in better health, improved mental and physical functioning, enhanced resistance to stress, a better sex life, and a host of other benefits.

FLAT EARTH SYNDROME

If the standard, conventional medical way of looking at things were enforced 100 percent, most of the effective treatments and preventive strategies we are now taking for granted would never have been adopted. New developments always take time before they're accepted, and there is always a group of people that energetically oppose any new developments that don't fit into their way of doing things.

Fortunately, there are as well a group of people who set the pace, who are dissatisfied with the status quo and who demand more. They want better methods of preventing illness, they want better food, they want to feel better and to perform better. Such people exist not only among nutritionists and nutritionally oriented physicians, but also among medical researchers and FDA officials.

But there will always be those who are afraid of change and who fight it with all their might, people who resist any ideas that tend to challenge or expand the standard ways of doing things. These people suffer from what we call the "flat earth syndrome." There are still people who believe the earth is flat, just as there are people who vehemently oppose the notion that you can prevent and treat illness with better nutrition and supplements.

THE CHOICE IS YOURS

You have a choice. You can wait until the evidence becomes overwhelming and accepted by even the most stubborn medical authorities. Or you can decide to try to do all that you can for yourself from available evidence.

NUTRITION NEWS TRAVELS WITH DEADLY SLOWNESS

A case in point. We have watched with fascination all the recent attention paid to calcium. The medical establishment and the news media have finally acknowledged that we need more calcium in our diets. But the "news" that a high calcium diet is needed to maintain the strength of our bones is not news at all. We—and a lot of other people—have known for more than a decade. The basic research has been published for more than a decade!

Are you prepared to wait another 10 years to discover all the health benefits of other vitamins, minerals, and our Beyond Vitamins supplements?

Another case, this one about a disease that was taking tens of thousands of lives. A physician, after much research and clinical experience, recommended a food supplement that he believed would prevent as well as cure the disease. To back him up, he also had evidence that in another country this disease had been eradicated nearly 200 years earlier —through the use of this same food supplement.

Do you know how long it was before this doctor's recommendations were finally adopted and the mounting death toll was stopped? It took 38 years.

The doctor was James Lind, the disease was scurvy, and the food supplement was vitamin C (from citrus fruit or juice). In 1757, England was at war, and yet more British sailors were dying from scurvy than from combat. And although Lind, a naval surgeon, recommended the use of citrus fruit to prevent scurvy (as the Dutch had discovered 200 years previously), the practice was not adopted until 38 years later, in 1795. Scurvy then disappeared from the British Navy.

More than 60 years later, however, the news of the benefits of citrus as a food supplement still hadn't helped people in the United States. As many as 15 percent of all Civil War deaths have been attributed to scurvy.

AND WE'RE STILL SUFFERING FROM IT

People in the United States are still suffering from scurvy, according to the *Journal of the American Medical Association.* Although the American Medical Association (AMA) tends to criticize nutritional supplements, the *Journal* of the AMA often contains some of the best evidence for taking them. In the February 8, 1985, issue (Vol. 253, No.6) it was reported that "scurvy is a disease that can mimic other more serious disorders . . . and because the clinical features of scurvy are no longer well appreciated, scorbutic patients are often extensively evaluated for other disorders."

In other words, most physicians believe that everyone gets all the vitamin C they need, so they fail to suspect scurvy when faced with the symptoms. The symptoms of scurvy can mimic the symptoms of cardiovascular disease, arthritis, infectious disorders, and many other common illnesses usually treated by means far more expensive than vitamin C supplementation. This article suggests that a lot of illness and unnecessary medical treatment might be prevented by making sure everyone got plenty of vitamin C in their diets.

Of course, if you read nutrition books and magazines 5, 10, 20, or even 30 years ago, the fact that millions of people are still suffering from vitamin C deficiency would not surprise you.

CAN WE GET ALL OUR VITAMINS AND MINERALS FROM OUR DIET?

Some people argue that we can get all the vitamins, minerals, and (after this book is published) Beyond Vitamins nutrients from our diets. Those who accept this argument say that's it's "unnatural" to take supplements, and if you just eat the right foods you will get all the nutrients you need. After all, our ancestors got along fine without supplements, didn't they?

Actually, they didn't. It's just a fantasy to think that things were better in the "good old days." And it's even more of a fantasy to think that we can return to the good old days if only we eat the right foods. Unfortunately, you can't find a natural food that isn't in some way tainted with the pollution of the twentieth century. Our bodies need help in dealing with that pollution.

On the average, we live a lot longer than our ancestors. Modern life stresses us in many ways, but our ancestors lived with many stresses. It's unreasonable to assume that because more of us are living longer than our ancestors that we are better off nutritionally. The things that killed them off are not the same things that are killing us off. And evidence continues to mount that the things that are sickening us are related to the inadequacies of our diet and the stresses of our modern life.

It is true that we need to eat more like our ancient ancestors did, because our bodies are biochemically set up to do best on the kinds of foods that we ate for millions of years, as we evolved. We may wear different clothes and zip around in cars and planes, but our bodies are still like the one million B.C. model.

THE BOTTOM LINE: WE WANT TO BE BETTER!

But beyond all, we really can't compare ourselves with our ancestors. The circumstances under which we live are so different that we may as well be living on a different planet. Our ancestors may or may not have sought out foods that were especially high sources of nutrients, although there is some evidence they did. It doesn't matter whether they did or not. What does matter is that *we* live in a polluted, dangerous world. Besides, not only do we want to survive, but we also want to be better than we were before. We want to perform better, achieve more, and live longer than our ancestors. And we know that increasing the nutrients in our diet will help us do that.

How do we know? Mostly from our own experience and from the many volumes of scientific evidence about the beneficial biological effects of all the individual nutrients in this book. The weight of this evidence suggests that providing more of certain nutrients will help us live longer, happier lives.

TAKING SUPPLEMENTS IS NATURAL

Besides, taking supplements *is* a natural act. It puts us more in step with nature. Let us explain: Modern life tends to cut us off from the flow of nature, the flow of matter and energy. Minerals and the molecules that make up vitamins and other nutrients are part of the flow of life through our bodies. But our processed food is so devoid of nutrients that is does little to maintain the flow. And even our natural food does not provide nutrients in the same concentrations as the same foods did 50, 100, or 1,000 years ago.

Taking nutritional supplements puts us more in touch

with nature by increasing the flow of life-giving minerals and nutritional molecules through our bodies. When the flow reaches optimum proportions, we are healthier, stronger, and happier than when the flow is weak—even if someone has incorrectly defined that impaired flow as "normal" or "adequate."

YOU CAN TAKE AN EVOLUTIONARY STEP RIGHT NOW

Evolutionary changes normally require thousands of years to take hold. Someday, there may be a race of humans that can live healthy, satisfying lives eating processed food, breathing filthy air, and drinking polluted water. Because we want to live healthy lives *now*, we're taking the evolutionary step of providing our bodies with the nutrients they need to stay fit.

But are we sure we're doing the right thing?

Yes, we are.

NUTRITION MAKES A BIG DIFFERENCE

Though most studies tend to focus on specific biochemical effects of individual supplements, there is one classic study about the long-term benefit of a general high-nutrient-density diet. From 1948 until 1954, Dr. Harold Chope kept health and diet records for almost 600 residents of San Mateo County, California. Dr. Chope was interested in finding out whether dietary levels of vitamin A, the B vitamins, and vitamin C had any relation to how long people lived and how free from disease they were.

Dr. Chope discovered some remarkable facts. A high-nutrient-density diet did, in fact, lengthen life and prevent disease. Four times as many people with low levels of vitamin C in their diet died during the study as did people with high levels. Diseases of the circulatory system, respiratory system, and nervous system were less common in people with high levels of vitamin A. And diseases of the circulatory system and digestive tract were less common in persons with high levels of vitamin C (*The American Journal of Clinical Nutrition*, Vol.23, N.3, pp.311–29).

Someday, someone will perform a similar experiment on a much grander scale. The diet and health records for thousands of people will be kept for several years and then analyzed, and all of the Beyond Vitamins supplements will be included. We're confident that such a study will find that supplements help us live longer; resist disease; improve our strength, stamina, and endurance; and, in general, make life fuller, as well as longer.

Here is just a single example of the kind of difference supplements can make.

Linda was a 42-year-old real estate agent beset with recurrent yeast infections. She also complained of nagging fatigue, which she overcame by sheer force of will. Although her symptoms were not drastically affecting her work, she was afraid her marriage was doomed. Because of the persistent vaginal itching and discharges that accompanied her yeast infection, she was rarely able to make love. Her husband was a patient, loving man who wanted to do all he could to help her get well. But after more than two years of going from doctor to doctor in search of a cure, both Linda and her husband were ready to believe that her symptoms were psychological, as several physicians suggested.

Linda told me that I (MR) was her last hope. If we couldn't control or reduce her symptoms, she and her husband were going to see a marriage counselor!

I took Linda's medical and dietary history. Aside from the fact that she and her husband were vegetarians, there didn't seem to be any extraordinary features. She ate practically no junk food, drank no coffee, and got plenty of exercise. She said she did not believe in taking supplements, preferring to get all her nutrients from her food.

Linda underwent the standard laboratory tests designed

to reveal nutritional deficiencies. I explained to her that these tests were useful and constantly becoming more sophisticated, but that the best guide to her nutritional status was the way she felt.

I had a suspicion of what was causing Linda's problems. But I waited until the tests came back, because I knew I would need them in order to convince her of a few things.

Sure enough, my hunch was correct. Linda's problem was caused by a deficiency of iron, and she was also deficient in a few other key immune nutrients. I had the results in black and white. Now all I had to do was convince her of what she needed to do to get better.

I began by telling Linda that she had several nutritional deficiencies. She tensed. I could tell she was going to resist what was coming. "I am committed to getting all of my nutrients from my food," she declared.

I confessed to her that although I was a nutritionally trained physician, I could not hope to design a better diet for her, one that would provide substantially more of the nutrients she was missing. As far as I could tell, her diet was providing much more than the Recommended Daily Allowance (RDA) of everything!

But, I explained, not nearly enough for her. Linda's personal requirements were apparently higher than most people's. That, coupled with the fact that our food supply wasn't supplying the levels of nutrients that the books said it did, was causing a shortfall in her nutritional status.

I told Linda that as much as I respected her right to eat whatever kind of diet she chose, her body had very real needs that did not respect her concepts. "You do have a choice, Linda. Either you eat substantially more food—or take some nutritional supplements. Since you're not underweight, I would expect that eating more food would result in a weight gain. My recommendation would be to take some nutritional supplements."

I told her that iron deficiency was among the most common deficiencies, and that one of its effects was to weaken the immune system against yeast infections. It also accounted for her fatigue.

Then I went on to explain how her tests had shown that she was also low in vitamin A, the B vitamins, zinc, and vitamin C. All of these nutrients are important for a healthy immune system.

Linda thought it over and agreed to try some supplements. I started her on a basic multivitamin-mineral supplement with iron. After two weeks, I broadened her program to include some of the Beyond Vitamins supplements described in this book.

Within a month, Linda reported that she felt stronger and had more energy. She still had some symptoms from her yeast infection, but these were improving. After two months, all symptoms of her yeast infection were gone. Linda asked me if she could reduce the number of supplements she was taking. I agreed that she could go back to her basic multivitamin-mineral with iron as long as she was free of yeast infections.

Linda reports back from time to time and tells me that she is doing just fine. Occasionally, during periods of increased stress, she has a brief recurrence of her yeast infection, which she deals with by going back to a full supplement program. She has learned to increase her supplements as a preventive measure during those periods. As far as her marriage is concerned, a marriage counselor is the last thing on her mind.

THE RDAS ARE A GOOD GUIDE—AND SO IS A WORLD MAP MADE IN 1491

There are only two groups of people for whom the RDAs are valuable: food processors and politicians. As a realistic nutritional guide for you or me, the RDAs are worthless. First of all, they bear very little relation to nutritional reality. Nature doesn't follow any committee's guidelines. Second, as unrealistically low as they are, few people are meeting them.

The RDAs are valuable to food processors because they

allow them to say that their products "supply 100 percent of the RDA for these essential vitamins and minerals." Because most of the nutritional value is processed out of food, it helps to have the standards set so low that even near-worthless foods can be advertised to "supply 100 percent." —100 percent of what? One hundred percent of what the committee decided was the amount we need. We're supposed to ignore the fact that a healthy portion of the committee is fortified with people who either work directly for the food industry or whose careers are indirectly supported by it.

A SMOKESCREEN FOR MALNUTRITION

The RDAs are valuable to politicians because they allow them to ignore widespread malnutrition in the United States and in other countries. They can report statistics such as "more than half of the population is obtaining a diet that supplies more than 70 percent of the RDA." The World Health Organization's RDAs are even lower than those for the United States. Many developing and long-since developed countries might be embarrassed if they had to report that a large proportion of their population was severely malnourished.

The fact that the U.S. RDAs are higher than the World Health Organization's is used to disguise the studies which have revealed that sizable portions of our population are eating diets that supply less than 70 percent of the RDA for certain vital nutrients, studies which report that: 51 percent are deficient in B_6, 42 percent in calcium, 39 percent in magnesium, 32 percent in iron, 31 percent in vitamin A, 26 percent in vitamin C, 17 percent in thiamine, 15 percent in B_{12}, and 12 percent in riboflavin (Pao, E.M., and Sharon Mickle, "Problem Nutrients in the United States," *Food Technology*, September 1981).

The Food and Nutrition Board, which sets the RDAs, has

recently been embroiled in arguments over whether or not to include in its deliberations the mountains of evidence that increased amounts of certain nutrients help prevent certain diseases. The evidence they're afraid to allow as evidence for the RDAs is exactly the kind of evidence we're providing in this book. We sympathize with the men and women on the Board. Can you imagine what would happen if the RDAs were suddenly raised to levels more in line with the amounts that we know will help promote health and prevent serious disease?

THE EVIDENCE IS CLEAR: WE AREN'T GETTING ENOUGH

Regardless of whether the RDAs ever reflect nutritional reality, the present food supply doesn't even supply the current RDAs! There is no scarcity of evidence that our diets aren't supplying the nutrients we need.

In one study, 49 percent of female and 15 percent of male teenagers were found to be consuming fewer than 4 mg. per day of pantothenic acid. (Nutritional Status Assessment, 3072).

A British study found that supplementation of women in the months before conception significantly reduced the number of birth defects, even among those who had previously given birth to babies with defects (*The Lancet*, June 15, 1985).

A Texas study found that college-aged women do not select a diet that supplies adequate amounts of B$_6$ or iron. More than 90 percent of the subjects selected diets inadequate in iron (*Nutr. Rep. In.*, Vol. 31, 1985, pp. 281–285.)

Washington State researchers examined the diets of female gymnasts and found that the young women selected diets that were inadequate in most B vitamins, iron, calcium, zinc, and magnesium. (*Journal of the American Dietetic Association*, Vol. 84, November 1984, pp. 1361–1363).

A study of adolescent women found that half were selecting diets supplying less than two-thirds of the RDA for B_6. Biochemical tests revealed that 20 percent of the young women had marginal B_6 status and 13 percent were frankly deficient (*Journal of the American Dietetic Association*, Vol. 85, No.1, January 1985, pp. 46–48).

A Utah study found that when pregnant women did not take pantothenic acid supplements, they had inadequate levels of the vitamin in their diet or their blood. This study was performed only to ascertain pantothenic acid status. It should not be interpreted to mean that pregnant women need only pantothenic acid supplements (*Journal of the American Dietetic Association*, Vol. 85, No. 2, February 1985, p. 192).

A year-long study found that adult men and women selected diets that were deficient in zinc and copper, supplying less than two-thirds of the RDA for these minerals (*The American Journal of Clinical Nutrition* 40, December 1984, pp. 1397–1403).

A similar study found that adult women were selecting diets that were universally deficient in iron (*The American Journal of Clinical Nutrition*, Vol. 40, December 1984, pp. 1393–1396).

The U.S. Department of Agriculture found that adult men and women tended to select diets that put them in negative balance for magnesium and calcium, meaning that they excreted more calcium than they took in—a sign that their bodies supplies of these minerals were being depleted (*The American Journal of Clinical Nutrition*, Vol. 40: December 1984, pp. 1368–1389).

Another USDA study found that higher-than-RDA levels of vitamin C served to increase blood levels of HDL cholesterol in men. HDL levels are thought to be protective against cardiovascular disease. The researchers concluded that this finding "may indicate that the optimal intake of vitamin C is higher than the RDA, especially for men." (*The American Journal of Clinical Nutrition*, Vol. 40, December 1984, p. 1338–1344).

A two-year survey of the diets of adult women found that 70 percent had diets that supplied less than 70 percent of the RDA—even with added supplements—of zinc and folic acid. About 30 percent had diets that supplied less than 70 percent of the RDAs for calcium and iron, and 40 percent had diets deficient in magnesium and vitamin B$_6$. (*Journal of the American Dietetic Association*, Vol. 84, September 1984, No. 9).

A Canadian study found that the risk of marginal deficiencies of vitamins A, C, E, and folic acid was greater in infants who did not receive supplements of these vitamins. Blood levels of these vitamins were in the area of marginal deficiency in unsupplemented infants and children (*Internat. J. Vit. Nutr. Res.* Vol. 55, 1985, pp. 205–216.)

Other studies have found American women's diets to be low in calcium, iron, magnesium, vitamin A, vitamin C, and B$_6$ (Pao, E.M. and S.J. Mickle. "Problem Nutrients in the United States" *Food Technology*, September 1981, pp. 60–79).

These are not isolated studies. These results continue to be reproduced in study after study across the country year after year. The subjects of the studies are neither poor nor underprivileged. They're just like you and me: They're not getting enough vital nutrition in their food.

It's no secret that we need more vitamins, minerals, and other nutrients than our diet provides. Although there are several special interests who want to keep the subject "controversial," the scientific evidence is solid. The median caloric intake for American men is about 1,800. For women it's 1,500. That means half of all American women are consuming fewer than 1,500 calories. A trained nutritionist would have a difficult time designing a day-to-day diet that would supply the RDA at that low level of food consumption. (Mark D. Hegsted, "Nationwide Food Consumption Survey—Implications," *Family Economics Review*, Spring, 1980, Dept. of Agriculture, Science and Education Administration, Beltsville, MD).

WHY DO MOST ANIMALS GET SUPPLEMENTS?

A curious fact: Why do you suppose food for animals is so highly supplemented? Animal feed usually supplies from 5 to 25 times the equivalent RDA for animals. Why? Because the people who produce animal feed recognize the benefit in high-density nutrition. Is it a coincidence that the amount of vitamin C supplied in monkey and guinea pig chow is similar to the amount that gorillas obtain in the wild and also to the amount Linus Pauling recommends for humans—and much, much higher than the RDA? (*Journal of Applied Nutrition*, Vol. 36, No. 2, 1984, pp. 163–170).

Does this evidence carry over and suggest that we're equally deficient in Beyond Vitamins supplements? We believe it does. Many Beyond Vitamins supplements are found in high-nutrient-density foods, foods which are fading from the modern diet. The deficiencies of Beyond Vitamins supplements could be even more severe and widespread, because processed foods are not "fortified" with any Beyond Vitamins nutrients.

THE MOST EXPENSIVE URINE IN THE WORLD ARGUMENT

This is one of our favorites. You've heard it: "People who take supplements have the most expensive urine in the world." The implication is that we're wasting our money because some of our supplements end up in the toilet.

The people who support this argument have a peculiar idea of human anatomy. They seem to believe that the parts of the body that can benefit from supplements stop somewhere short of the excretory organs.

If you want your supplements to benefit your entire body —even your organs of elimination, you're going to have to get used to the idea that some of the nutrients are going to wind up in your sweat, urine, stool, and mucus. That's not a waste. Far from it! Nutrients that are excreted help to prevent illness on the way out of the body as well as while inside it. For example, we know that the urine of smokers contains mutagenic compounds (*Carcinogenisis*, Vol. 5 No. 11, 1984, pp. 1523–1524). We also know that vitamin C can detoxify mutagenic compounds in the urine as well as in the feces. So is it really a waste to have vitamin C in our urine?

Are people wasting money on supplements? Hardly. Americans spend about $3 billion for supplements every year. We spend $20 billion on tobacco and $40 billion on alcoholic beverages. But even these amounts pale against the total bill for medical care, which is in the neighborhood of $400 billion and growing. Rather, the evidence suggests that a little money spent on good nutrition can save a lot on medical care (Gallo, Anthony F. "Food Spending and Income," *National Food Review*, USDA Economic Research Service, Winter 1982; *Medical Tribune*, Vol. 24 (No. 19) p. 1, 1983).

THE EVIDENCE IS SOLID

Some critics acknowledge that there is "some evidence" that supplements are helpful, but dismiss it by saying that it's "suggestive rather than conclusive." The fact is that most medical practice is based on evidence that is gathered and reported according to the very same standards as scientific research on nutrition. Nutritional evidence tends to be even more reliable, if only because it is less subject to the current fashions of drug and surgical therapy. Scientists and clinicians have been gathering evidence about the effects of diet on health for much, much longer than they have been studying the latest drug or surgical techniques.

FILE THIS UNDER: "DON'T DO AS I DO, DO AS I SAY"

Dieticians are often the most vocal critics of supplements. After all, they are trained to design food programs that will supply adequate nutrition. It's very important to their professional image to maintain the idea that we can, after all, get all the nutrients we need from our food. It's also important because many professional dieticians are trained in programs that are supported in part by the processed food industry, and their food programs often contain high concentrations of processed foods.

Because it's so important for them to enforce this view, dieticians are lobbying in many states for laws that would prohibit the sale of nutritional supplements except by a dietician or through a physician's prescription.

Thus, it's quite interesting to discover, thanks to a Washington State survey or more than 900 dieticians, that nearly 60 percent admitted that they took some form of nutritional supplement. The most commonly used supplements were multivitamins and minerals and vitamin C. According to the authors of the study, a higher percentage of dieticians (60 percent) use supplements than the general population (54 percent).

The authors took pains to apologize for the dietician's personal departure from the party line: "Traditionally, dieticians maintain the view that sound dietary practices will support nutritional health for the vast majority of the healthy population. They are aware, however, of provocative new research and cognizant of the life-style and other characteristics of individuals which warrant the use of specific nutritional supplements."

Welcome to the club, ladies and gentlemen. It's nice to

know that dieticians have feet of clay just like the rest of us. Now, if they'd only admit that we have the same rights to look at that "provocative new research" and make up our minds how to supplement our diets as well (*Journal of the American Dietetic Association*, Vol. 84, No. 7, p. 795).

We've written this book to help you bring the fruits of that provocative new research into your own life. We hope you'll start making use of this new information to build a healthier, more satisfying life.

Index